Peripheral Manipulation

By the same author

Vertebral
Manipulation

Peripheral Manipulation

Second Edition

G. D. Maitland,

AUA, FCSP, MAPA

Part-time Senior Lecturer and Clinical Tutor for the 'Graduate Diploma in Advanced Manipulative Therapy' within the School of Physiotherapy of the South Australian Institute of Technology, Adelaide

Butterworths

London · Boston · Durban · Singapore · Sydney · Toronto · Wellington

First published 1970
Reprinted 1974
Reprinted 1976
Second Edition, 1977
Reprinted 1978
Reprinted 1979
Reprinted 1980
Reprinted 1981
Reprinted 1983
Reprinted 1984

ISBN 0 407 35672 X

© Butterworth & Co (Publishers) Ltd, 1977

British Library Cataloguing in Publication Data

Maitland, Geoffrey Douglas
   Peripheral manipulation. – 2nd ed.
   1. Joints   2. Manipulation (Therapeutics)
   I. Title
   616.7′2′0622   RC932   77–30018

ISBN 0 407 35672 X

Photoset by Butterworths Litho Preparation Department
Printed and bound in Great Britain by Biddles Ltd, Guildford and King's Lynn

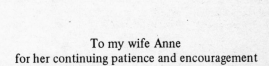

To my wife Anne
for her continuing patience and encouragement

Foreword

Mobilization and manipulation of joints by physiotherapists are very important subjects. At present the techniques to be used and the indications for their use are being discussed extensively, and undoubtedly they will be subjected to a steadily increasing thorough assessment. Everyone wants to know how much to do and when. Consequently it is no surprise that Geoffrey Maitland has been persuaded by his colleagues to write about peripheral joints, as a companion to his previous book *Vertebral Manipulation*.[1] Although he is most widely known for his work on the spine, when he came to England on a lecture tour in 1966 it was very noticeable how often he was engaged in discussions with physiotherapists on the best methods of mobilizing peripheral joints. Physiotherapists everywhere will be delighted that he has written this further book.

In the past there have been too many hasty judgments and firmly entrenched views on this subject, particularly whenever the word 'manipulation' has been used. Exaggerated claims and intolerant condemnation have been equally common; and both have held up the development and assessment of mobilization and manipulation that are so badly needed. Every physiotherapist knows that the least possible force should be used to produce the desired result; and yet some doctors have implied that these manœuvres are always forceful and liable to cause damage. Others have condemned repeated gentle passive mobilization, but have been content to prescribe vigorous active exercises or to perform forceful manipulation under anaesthesia for the same conditions. Such judgments are unfair.

[1] Maitland, G. D. (1977). *Vertebral Manipulation.* London; Butterworths

This book deserves to be read with respect, and so do the other books by physiotherapists on this subject which will undoubtedly follow. Geoffrey Maitland is well aware of the limitations of our knowledge and he is always modest in describing his results. Undoubtedly he is putting forward his own views with humility, hoping to promote discussion so that others can improve on his own suggestions. The question he raises is simple enough; if a patient has a stiff or painful shoulder, knee, ankle, temperomandibular joint or elbow, is it sufficient for a physiotherapist to apply heat or ice, or teach a regimen of active exercises; or may she need to apply a gentle passive movement, a nudge at the extreme of range, perhaps in a direction not normally followed by the joint when moving under voluntary control? Unfortunately it is not easy to give a firm answer, or to decide on the best techniques or their indications. Controlled trials are obviously needed; but it might be many years before they produce adequate answers, and consequently it is essential to achieve an interim assessment based on clinical judgment and experience. To do this, physiotherapists must improve their techniques and define them more precisely; and doctors must spend more time watching to see exactly what is done and observing the results. In the meantime this book clearly expresses the views of a very experienced physiotherapist, and undoubtedly it will lead to much thought and discussion.

D. A. Brewerton

Preface to Second Edition

Since the first edition of this book in 1970 there have been rapid changes in attitude towards manipulative treatment as applied to the spine. Manipulation is now accepted fairly generally as a routine part of medicine. More and more courses are being conducted by and for doctors of medicine and physiotherapists and the standards attained by these courses are steadily improving year by year. In Australia the States of Western Australia and South Australia are conducting 12-month full-time postgraduate courses leading to a 'Graduate Diploma in Manipulative Therapy'; other countries too are constantly upgrading their undergraduate and postgraduate trainings in this field.

With the acceptance of manipulation in relation to the spine, it is now being realized that mobilizing techniques have a particular part to play in the treatment of peripheral joints. Stretching peripheral joints which are limited in range is common practice for physiotherapists but only now are they realizing that gentle oscillatory passive movements can be used to relieve joint pain. To most physiotherapists and even to some manipulative physiotherapists this is a new concept. The application of passive treatment technique needs to be seen to be appreciated.

The theory and practice is essentially the same as for the vertebral column. However, because of the multiple joints between two vertebrae and the presence of the spinal cord, vertebral artery and nerve roots, treatment for the vertebral column is far more complex.

When treating peripheral joints, the factors to guide treatment are range of movement, pain with movement, stiffness due to contracted soft tissue structures or adhesions, etc. and muscle spasm.

I am greatly indebted to Mr Brian Edwards BSc, BAppSc (Physio)

PREFACE TO SECOND EDITION

for the constructive criticism and considerable help he has afforded me. My wife has again produced more drawings of techniques. Without her help and her supporting encouragement this edition could not have been written.

Adelaide   G. D. Maitland

Preface to First Edition

Treatment of painful peripheral joints by passive movement has become almost a forgotten art among physiotherapists. In the present era active exercise, combined with heat or cold therapy, is the popular and established approach. Passive movement is not routinely used because in the past its techniques have been used too strongly, causing the patient unnecessary discomfort and sometimes aggravating the condition.

Hesitation on the part of doctors and physiotherapists to use passive movement arises from a lack of understanding of how and when to apply gentle techniques, and of their effectiveness. Physiotherapists, inexperienced in handling painful joints passively, may have inadvertently aggravated the pain and thus wrongly concluded that passive movement should not be used. This conclusion is unfortunate; when precise physical signs of joint disturbance can be determined, quicker and better results may be achieved using passive movement guided by the signs. Often quite gentle techniques can be used.

Many books have been written about manipulation of peripheral joints. Among these are important contributions by Dr Cyriax[1] and Drs James[2] and John Mennell[3]. Dr Cyriax's work is particularly notable for the presentation of accurate methods of examination. The treatment techniques he outlines are those of the stronger type, some of

[1] Cyriax, J. (1965). *Textbook of Orthopaedic Medicine*. Vol. II, 7th edn. London; Baillière Tindall

[2] Mennell, James (1952). *Science and Art of Joint Manipulation*. Vol. II. London; Churchill

[3] Mennell, John McM. (1964). *Joint Pain*. Boston; Little Brown & Co (1965) London; Churchill

which require the assistance of physiotherapists. Dr John Mennell (1964) continues the work of his father, Dr James Mennell (1952), who stressed the importance of accessory movement (or, in his own terminology, 'joint play').

Even with these books, and others written by lay manipulators there are still several facets of the field of passive movement treatment which are not covered. There are occasions when patients are referred for physiotherapy with joint disorders which require techniques not previously described, or when the reasons for choosing particular amplitudes and positions in the range have not previously been described or related to the examination findings of the joint disorders.

The purpose of this book is to present techniques for all peripheral joints, to discuss in detail the relevant parts of examination by passive movement, and to relate the method of applying the techniques to the examination findings.

Most people think of passive movement treatment as a stretching process to increase the range of movement of a stiff joint. However, the application of passive movement to painful peripheral joints is far wider than this. *Its use in the treatment of joint pain, whether the range of movement is limited or not, has not been appreciated.* This subject has not been treated in any other text published and possibly may not have been considered before. For this reason alone the following text is necessary to fill a gap in the physical treatment of joint pain.

Although some of the techniques will be similar to those published by others, many will be different, and some of the moving parts for which techniques are described have not been presented before. Also, some of the movements described for certain joints have not been presented before.

Diagnosis will not be discussed in this book as this is the province of the medical practitioner. However, when he refers a patient, very careful examination of joint movement must be undertaken by the physiotherapist. The findings will guide the choice of technique and the style of movement to be used (i.e. small amplitude, large amplitude, avoiding pain or moving into pain), and the range in which it is performed. The findings also act as guides for the assessment of progress.

When any new form of treatment becomes popular, people tend to think only about the new techniques; the idea being that once the techniques are learned, nothing remains but to apply them to patients. If this idea is carried out by numerous people, it follows that standards of treatment fall, results are poor, and consequently the treatment method lapses. This idea of solely learning techniques and applying them indiscriminately is totally inadequate. For this reason considerable space in the ensuing text is given to minute examination detail and to the ways in which the techniques should be applied to the findings. The process may seem tedious at first and may even emphasize the points which seem too trivial to mention. However, this depth of detail is designed to prevent misunderstanding of the reasons for the application of the techniques. Also as a musculoskeletal disorder may present different joint signs at different stages of development of the complaint, it is essential that examination of the joint signs be carried out in detail. Different joint signs require different treatment techniques.

In the chapter on Examination appreciation of the various factors which constitute the joint signs determined by passive movement tests is discussed. In the appendices 'movement diagrams' have been offered as the best method at present available for teaching this appreciation. The 'movement diagram' has also been used in the chapter on Treatment to express more clearly the relationship between passive movement used in treatment and the clinical signs. The concept of a 'movement diagram' was evolved by Miss J—M. Ganne, MCSP, MAPA, DipTP, and further developed in an article jointly written by Miss Jennifer Hickling, MCSP and the author, published in the *Journal of the Chartered Society of Physiotherapy*[1] and the *Australian Journal of Physiotherapy*[2]. Thanks are due to Miss Hickling and to the Editors of both journals for permitting part of the article to be reproduced in this book.

Dr D. A. Brewerton, MD, FRCP, has provided an invaluable medical approach to the many aspects of passive movement treatment, and I am grateful to him for his contribution. Much needs to be said about attitudes to and prejudices against this form of treatment which cannot properly be said by a physiotherapist, and I am very pleased to have Dr Brewerton's willing support and I thank him sincerely. Many amendments regarding presentation were made to the text as it evolved and Mrs J. Trott, Miss Patricia Trott, AVA, Grad. Dip. Manip. Ther., MAPA, MCSP, and Miss M. J. Hammond, AUA, MAPA, MCSP, Dip.TP, have been patient, helpful and encouraging. The illustrations drawn by my wife more than achieve their purpose. They clearly and simply illustrate the text and avoid the distractions often present with photographs. I am especially grateful for her helpfulness and suggestions throughout the project. Without the willing help of the many people who carried out typing, modelling, and drawing of graphs, the book could not have been completed and I extend to them my grateful thanks.

Adelaide   G. D. Maitland
                                                                           1970

[1] Hickling, J. and Maitland, G. D. (1970). 'Abnormalities in passive movement: diagrammatic representation.' *J. chart. Soc. Physiother.* **56**, 105

[2] Hickling, J. and Maitland, G. D. (1970). 'Abnormalities in passive movement: diagrammatic representation.' *Aust. J. Physiother.* XVI, 13

Contents

Part I THEORY

1 Manipulation: Definition and Role   3

2 Examination   7

3 Principles of Technique   28

4 Treatment: Method and Assessment   32

5 Treatment: Application of Techniques   45

Part II JOINT TECHNIQUES AND MANAGEMENT

6 Shoulder Girdle   61

7 Upper Limb   121

8 Lower Limb   203

9 Other Joints and Structures   315

Part III APPLICATION

10 Recording   333

Appendix 1   338

Appendix 2   348

Index   355

Part I

THEORY

1 Manipulation: Definition and Role

DEFINITION

The term 'manipulation' can be used loosely in medicine to mean passive movement of any kind. As used in this text it can be divided into the following.

1. MOBILIZATION

Mobilizations are passive movements performed in such a way (particularly in relation to the speed of the movements) that at all times they are within the control of the patient so that he can prevent the movement if he so chooses. Two main types of movement are:

(a) passive oscillatory movements, two or three per second, of small or large amplitude, and applied anywhere in a range of movement;

(b) sustained stretching with tiny amplitude oscillations at the limit of the range.

These oscillatory movements may consist of the joint's accessory movements or its physiological movements. Physiological movements are those which the patient can carry out actively. Accessory movements are movements which a person cannot perform himself but which can be performed on him by someone else. For example, a person cannot rotate the metacarpophalangeal joint of his index finger but somebody else can rotate it for him. Therefore rotation of the metacarpophalangeal joint is an accessory movement.

The movements referred to in (a) and (b) above may be performed while the joint surfaces are held distracted or compressed. Distraction is the keeping apart of the opposing joint surfaces and compression means that the joint surfaces are squeezed together. Both positions are used in treatment.

2. MANIPULATION

There are two procedures which can be termed manipulation.

(a) Manipulation is a sudden movement or thrust, of small amplitude, performed at a speed which renders the patient powerless to prevent it.

(b) Manipulation under anaesthesia (MUA) is a medical procedure performed with the patient under anaesthesia and used to stretch a joint to restore a full range of movement by breaking adhesions. The procedure is not a sudden forceful thrust as mentioned in the preceding paragraph but is done as a steady and controlled stretch. This procedure can also be performed on the conscious patient.

If during treatment using the 'mobilizing' technique as described in 1 (b) above, adhesions are torn the mobilizing technique may then be classed as a manipulation even though a sudden thrust has not been used.

The 35th Edition of *Gray's Anatomy*[1], and particularly the section on Arthrology (pages 389–471), is among the best references relating to current knowledge of joint structure and function. Information fundamental to examination of joint disorders and treatment by passive movement is given; the bibliography and diagrams are excellent. It is important that physiotherapists treating joint disorders by passive movement be well versed in musculoskeletal anatomy, in the principles of movement at each joint, in the neurophysiology related to pain with joint movement, and in the part played by muscle spasm.

ROLE

Mobilization and manipulation show to best effect when directed at mechanical problems for which they perform three main roles.

1.   Restoring structures within a joint to their normal positions or pain-free positions so as to allow a full-range painless movement.

[1] *Gray's Anatomy* (1973). 35th Edition. London; Longman

If a patient has a damaged joint, such as a tear of the medial meniscus of the knee or temporomandibular joint, he will have a restricted range of movement which will be painful in some directions. Passive movement aims to alter the position of the meniscus so that the range of movement of the joint becomes full and pain free. When pain-free movement has been restored, the next step is to prevent recurrences by exercising to increase the power, the endurance and the speed with which the muscles can contract to control the movements.

2.   Stretching a stiff painless joint to restore range.

Passive movement techniques can be used to stretch a stiff pain-free joint in order to improve the range until it reaches the stage of being functional once more. The movements used should be those described in *Gray's Anatomy,* that is, treatment movements which include the spin, roll, and slide normal for that joint. There are other movements described in the text which are used to increase range. They should all be done as small, strong oscillatory movements performed at the rate of two or three per second. They will provide the manipulator with more accurate 'feel' of the resistance than would be possible with a sustained stretching technique.

3.   Relieving pain by using special techniques.

A patient may have considerable joint pain which limits his active movement, although there is no loss of passive range. In other words, if the examiner were prepared to ignore the patient's pain, and press on regardless, he would find the range of movement full in all directions though obviously they would be extremely painful. Mobilization has a definite part to play in the treatment of these painful joints.

With these joint disorders there is usually a degree of inflammation the cause of which is not always evident. There may be an outside factor causing it, for example rheumatoid arthritis or its variants, or there may be a mechanical irritating origin. This second group can be successfully treated by special passive movement techniques. If the mechanical treatment eliminates the mechanical irritating cause the patient loses his pain.

A patient may have more than one cause for an inflammatory reaction in a joint. For example, it is possible that a patient may have active rheumatoid arthritis producing inflammatory reaction, superimposed upon which a mechanical factor may be provoking further inflammatory reaction. If this is so, passive movement treatment can effect a degree of improvement commensurate with the extent of the mechanical cause.

Frequently at a first consultation it is impossible to determine whether or not a combination of factors is causing the painful reaction. However, if a short trial of controlled passive movement is administered it is possible to determine, in retrospect by assessment, the extent of the mechanical cause. If the treatment lessens the patient's pain and improves range then at least part of the patient's pain must have been mechanical in origin. However, if there is no improvement, there is no mechanical factor involved.

If a patient has an active osteoarthritis in a joint, mobilization will not improve the pain. However, if the diagnosis is osteoarthrosis, passive movement treatment should be a foremost consideration.

Most of the patients referred by doctors to physiotherapists for treatment of musculoskeletal problems seek help because of pain rather than stiffness. The joints should be tested for range and pain, and the muscles should be tested for strength and pain. If the examination is carried out correctly it will be found that most musculoskeletal problems have two components, a pain component and a stiffness component. Spasm may also be present and this may cloud the assessment, particularly if it prevents movement early in the range.

These components, or 'joint signs' in musculoskeletal disorders must be recognized and assessed independently. All physiotherapists have treated patients who have a stiff painless joint. They will also have treated patients who have pain associated with the stiffness. However, it is surprising how few physiotherapists recognize the group of patients who have painful joints which are not limited by any stiffness. It is important to be aware that such patients exist and that they can be treated by special passive movement techniques. When the concept of treating the pain component is understood, accepted and used, then treatment by manipulation can be utilized to its fullest extent.

2 Examination

When a patient with skeletal pain consults his doctor, the examination includes many tests which do not concern us here. However, if this patient is then referred for physiotherapy, the minute details of joint examination immediately become the physiotherapist's concern.

Although physical examination of posture, deformity and muscle power and assessment of other joints are important the detail of their examination will be omitted from the following discussion so that emphasis can be placed on the examination directly concerned with treatment by passive movement.

SUBJECTIVE EXAMINATION

The area, nature and behaviour of the patient's pain are the first details required.

In the search for the area of pain the findings should be exact, as these form the foundation on which the examination is built. If the area overlies a joint, the patient should be asked specifically if his pain is 'within' the joint, if necessary grasping the joint firmly, surrounding it while asking if the pain is 'deep inside'. It should be borne in mind that there may be more than one site of pain. For example, a patient may have a painful foot which causes pain and makes him limp. Though he may say in answer to the initial question that his pain is in his foot, more detailed interrogation may reveal that he has three sites of pain: one along the medial side of his foot, a second area along the lateral border of the foot, and a third site which he describes as being through and inside his ankle. Failure to ascertain such detail may lessen the effectiveness of examination, assessment and treatment.

Any areas of paraesthesia or anaesthesia should be marked on the body chart used to outline the areas of pain.

In relation to the 'behaviour' of the pain the patient should be asked to describe whether his pain is sharp, dull, throbbing, constant, variable or intermittent, and whether all areas of the pain occur simultaneously or whether different actions reproduce different pains (Table 2.1).

Table 2.1

Initial questions before asking the more direct questions

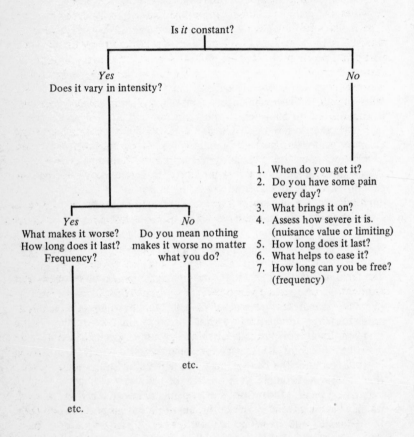

It is essential to know which is the main area of pain and what particular movements provoke it; if the joint is painful while at rest, if the resting pain is caused by some mechanical degree of stretch or compression affecting the joint, or whether by an active inflammatory process. If the joint is painful only when moved or exercised, the offending movements must be determined and the differences in the various directions of movement appreciated. Furthermore, it must be determined whether it is pain or stiffness which is of greater concern to the patient.

Pain can behave in so many different ways. However, there are two aspects which are commonly not appreciated. The first is that the patient may be able to carry out a day's activity with minimal inconvenience but finds that his pain develops *after* he stops these activities. A second variation can be that the pain only develops after a particular position has been adopted and maintained for some considerable period. It may develop following the sustaining of only one particular position or it may follow several different positions. A further example is evinced where a joint has been comfortably kept in a particular position for a length of time, then on moving from this position sudden sharp pain occurs. It may subside immediately, possibly leaving the patient pain free.

If the pain varies in any way (for example in area or intensity) an attempt should be made to find out which particular activities provoke the pain and how long the increased symptoms take to subside. If the patient's pain is only intermittent, its frequency and duration should also be determined.

'Behaviour' of the symptoms is important because the physiotherapist must know how and why the pain varies throughout a 24 hour period.

These differences of pain pattern must have some significance in relation to diagnosis but it is doubtful whether anyone as yet knows the reasons for the different patterns, and unfortunately there are physiotherapists who are unaware that pain can behave in so many ways. This leads to incomplete examination followed in turn by an incomplete understanding of the patient's problem.

When the pain is aggravated by movements it is helpful to ask the patient to demonstrate how he is restricted by the pain or stiffness. It is also useful to know if there are any positions he can adopt which relieve the symptoms.

'Irritability' is determined by relating the vigour of an activity which causes pain, firstly to the degree of pain which ensues, and then to the length of time taken for this increased pain to subside to its usual level. Such assessment is necessary to avoid excessive examination. Two examples may provide useful comparisons. Firstly, a school-teacher with shoulder pain is unable to write more than a few lines on the lower part of the blackboard without experiencing moderate pain which continues for more than an hour. This joint condition is irritable: it takes very little activity to cause considerable pain which takes a long time to subside. For this reason the patient should not be subjected to prolonged examination of painful movements because of the inevitable exacerbation. Treatment by passive movement in this instance must be gentle and the amplitude of movements used should be small. A second example is a patient who notices sharp momentary shoulder pain only if he mis-hits a drive at golf, or sustains similar jarring. This condition is not irritable and it is likely that, in order to determine the joint signs by which treatment can be guided, examination of his passive movements would need to be taken to the limit of the range and the various movements tested in finer detail and with greater strengths than with the first-mentioned patient. Also, treatment would probably require more vigour than the first patient's shoulder could tolerate.

'Irritability' has two other valuable uses. Firstly, assessment of joint-irritability provides details by which progress can be assessed from treatment to treatment. For example, if a patient at his initial interview says that, after sitting for half an hour it takes him two or three steps to get going again because of stiffness in his knee and at a later stage in treatment reports that after going to the theatre he was able to get out of his seat without difficulty, then obviously he has made some degree of progress. During the treatment, discussion of the progress being made can benefit both physiotherapist and patient. Assessment forms a vital role in treatment and will be discussed later.

The other reason for assessing joint-irritability lies in its relation to treatment. This will be considered later, as it has an important bearing on the type of movement chosen for a technique.

Details regarding the history of the present condition and any previous condition from which the patient may have been suffering, and which may bear relevance to the present condition, should be ascertained. The history (Table 2.2) of the patient's condition will indicate the diagnosis and also provide facts on which the prognosis and possibility of recurrence can be assessed. Knowing the precise movement which caused an injury can also have an important bearing on the examination and treatment. It should be ascertained whether the patient considers his symptoms are improving, worsening or static. As 'assessment' is the fulcrum about which the whole treatment programme is conducted, the importance of minute details regarding the patient's symptoms and their variations can be appreciated.

Routinely, a patient should be questioned regarding his general health and whether any particular tablets are being taken so that their possible effect may be appreciated and any dangers to treatment revealed.

Table 2.2

Present history

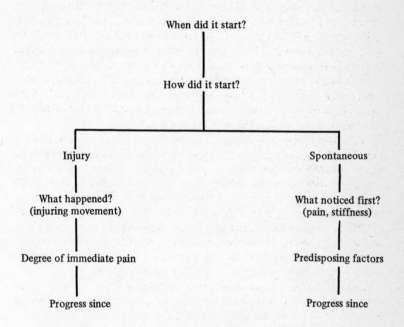

When did it start?

How did it start?

Injury

Spontaneous

What happened?
(injuring movement)

What noticed first?
(pain, stiffness)

Degree of immediate pain

Predisposing factors

Progress since

Progress since

1. Relate severity of incident to degree of disability for comparability (serious pathology)
2. History of local pain compared with history of referred pain
3. Progress over initial period until 'levelling off' of symptoms

Previous history

1. Related to this joint
2. Related to relevant joints
   (a) Other peripheral joints
   (b) Vertebral column

Table 2.3 summarizes what needs to be known and the sequence used during the subjective examination.

Table 2.3
Subjective Examination

Area

Is the disorder one of pain, stiffness or both?
Record on the 'body chart'
1. area and depth of pain, indicating areas of greatest intensity and stating type of symptoms
2. paraesthesia and anaesthesia
3. Check associated areas, i.e.
    (a) of vertebral column
    (b) of joints 'above and below' the lesion
    (c) other relevant joints

Behaviour of symptoms
1. When are they present or when do they fluctuate? constant, intermittent—frequency
2. Any pain at night? Need to get up because of it? Able to lie on it? (Is the night pain for mechanical reasons or inflammatory?)
3. On first rising c.f. end of day
4. What aggravates, what eases?
5. Functional limitations (dominance of pain or stiffness)

Special questions
1. General health, relevant weight loss
2. What tablets are being taken for this and other conditions? (steroids, pain-killers, anti-inflammatory drugs)

History
1. of this attack
2. Previous history
3. Are the symptoms worsening or improving?
4. Any previous treatment? Effect?
5. Any contraindications?

HIGHLIGHT MAIN FINDINGS WITH ASTERISKS

Planning the examination

PLANNING THE EXAMINATION

From the point of view of teaching it is helpful if the student completes a planning sheet (Table 2.4) before commencing the objective examination. By committing her thoughts and plans regarding the objective examination to paper, the novice helps the supervisor to follow her deliberations and thus to guide, correct and assist her.

Table 2.4
Planning the Examination

A The sources of the pain
    1. Name as the *possible* sources of *any part* of the patient's pain *every* joint
    and muscle which must be examined

Joints which lie under the painful area	*Joints* which refer pain into the area	*Muscles* which lie under the painful area

    2. Are you going to do a *Neurological* examination? *Yes/No*
    3. List joints 'above and below' the lesion which should be checked

B Influence of pain and pathology on examination
    1. Is pain 'severe'? *Yes/No*
    2. Does the subjective examination suggest an easily irritable disorder?
      Local pain   *Yes/No*   *Referred pain*   *Yes/No*
    Give the example
    Part (*i*) Activity causing pain ....
    Part (*ii*) Severity of pain so caused...
    Part (*iii*) Duration before pain subsides..
    3. Does the 'nature' of the disorder indicate caution? *Yes/No*
      (*i*) pathology (osteoporosis, RA etc.)
      (*ii*) easy to cause bouts
      (*iii*) imminent nerve root compression

C The kind of examination
    1. Do you think you would need to be gentle or moderately firm with
    your examination of movements?
    2. Do you expect a comparable sign { to be easy / or / to be hard } to find?
    3. Do you think you will be treating pain, resistance or weakness?

D Associated examination
    1. What associated factors must be examined
      (*a*) Reasons why the joint or muscle has become painful?
      (*b*) The effect of the disorder on the muscular control?
      (*c*) Why the joint or muscle pain *may* recur?

Reference to the planning sheet shows four sections. Section A refers to the structures which need to be examined as the cause of the disorder. Section B provides facts relating to the patient's symptoms which should guide the therapist in knowing how these symptoms are likely to behave as a reaction to the first day's examination test movements and treatment. Section C requires the student to decide the strength with which test movements need to be performed and to show how easy or difficult the important test signs will be to find. In other words, if a patient has a mild ache generally in his foot following a 10-mile walk then all the answers to the questions in Section B will lead the physiotherapist to the conclusion that her examination techniques will need to be 'moderately vigorous', thus avoiding a too-gentle examination routine which ends by revealing nothing. Similarly it also avoids doing too-vigorous examination techniques on a patient who has considerable pain and who would thus be subjected to exacerbation. Section D is self-explanatory. It is a second aspect of examination directed towards preventing recurrences rather than determining the painful structures. For example, a patient may have sprained his ankle badly. Sections A, B and C on the planning sheet will relate directly to treating the damaged structure, restoring range and thereby eliminating the pain. A separate and important aspect to the examination is directed towards preventing recurrences. Here section D of the planning comes into force. In the example above it relates directly to determining muscle weakness around the ankle from the point of view of its power and its speed of stabilizing action and to determining any other abnormalities which may lead to, or precipitate a recurrence.

OBJECTIVE EXAMINATION

Before any movements are tested actively, the physiotherapist should have a clear appreciation of the irritability of the joint disorder to know whether to limit test movements and so avoid exacerbation. If the joint-irritability is high, it is far wiser to spread the examination over more than one visit, leaving the less important details of examination until later.

Treatment by passive movement is based on the examination findings of the joint's movements in each direction. An assessment of the patient's active movements should be made to ascertain his willingness and ability to move, and to gain measurements on which future assessments can be made.

'Quick tests' (i.e. full-range active antigravity movements) should be done with the patient standing and the result of these will determine the requisite extent of the examination to follow. For example, if the patient has a hip, knee or ankle problem he should be asked to squat as far as possible. The degree of his disability will be quickly and clearly shown. If he is able to squat fully with minimal discomfort then the physiotherapist will have to examine joint movement quite vigorously if she is to find abnormalities. The relevant tests for each joint will be described in the text.

When examining joint movement the primary aim is to find a 'comparable sign' at an 'appropriate joint'.

A joint sign refers to any facet of movement of a joint which is abnormal. When dealing with musculoskeletal problems these abnormal findings will be stiffness, pain, or muscle spasm. A 'comparable' joint sign refers to combinations of pain, stiffness and spasm which the examiner finds on examination and considers to be comparable with the patient's symptoms. In other words, not all joint signs are relevant because they are not 'comparable' to the disorder. Also, it is quite common to find minor joint signs at an appropriate joint which are not comparable to the patient's disability. Such examination would reveal only mild pain and any stiffness present would be minimal.

Not only must the joint signs be comparable with the patient's disability they must also be in an 'appropriate joint'. In other words, there may be stiffness and pain on passive flexion of the metatarso-phalangeal joint of the big toe yet the patient's complaint may be pain felt anterior to the ankle joint. Obviously the joint signs found at the big toe are not in an 'appropriate joint'.

The aim of examining movements is to find one or more **comparable** 'signs' in an **appropriate** joint or joints.

Finding a comparable sign is not always easy and signs which may seem comparable at the first treatments, may prove to be otherwise. This may be so if the patient does not improve with treatment. Under these circumstances re-examination should be carried out with careful stronger test movements in an endeavour to find different signs which prove comparable. Having found such a sign and made use of it in treatment, the patient's symptoms and signs should improve. As improvement occurs, comparable signs may change and a new comparable sign may become evident. These changes of comparable signs will require changes in treatment techniques.

ACTIVE MOVEMENTS

As the first step in assessing a patient's active movements it is rewarding to ask what movements he can do at the moment which cause pain or show up his disability. If the physiotherapist then makes use of what the patient demonstrates, clear information is immediately gained.

While the joint is at rest and before carrying out any test movements of the joint the patient should be asked if he has any pain. The joint should then be moved in a particular direction until pain is first felt, or, if the joint has some degree of pain while at rest, the patient should be asked to move to the point where pain starts to increase. This range should then be noted and recorded by the physiotherapist.

If the joint-irritability assessed during the subjective examination indicates that exacerbation is unlikely to occur, the patient should then be asked to move the joint into the painful range as far as possible. Changes in the severity or area of the pain with the further movement should be noted and recorded together with the range at which pain started and the range which proved to be the limit of the patient's active movement.

If the subjective irritability and the severity of the pain permit, the patient should repeatedly move the part from the starting position to the limit of the range while the physiotherapist watches for abnormalities in the normal rhythm to determine in which individual joint the fault lies. It is obvious that such a test of the knee or elbow will reveal less than a test of the foot or shoulder where many joints work in harmony.

Sometimes it is necessary to include speed in the test movement to find abnormalities in the rhythm, when none are evident if the joint is moved at a normal speed. The speed of the test movement may then reveal abnormal rhythm and may also provoke and reproduce pain which otherwise would be missed.

All movements of a joint are assessed and if it is felt that a movement is full range and painless, a moderate degree of pressure is then applied at the limit of the range to assess whether the movement is in fact full range and painless. The pressure should not be excessive but applied with full appreciation of the age and general condition of the patient. Of equal importance, the over-pressure must not be too light. This is an essential test because frequently a patient considers his movements are normal when in fact there is some pain or restriction if over-pressure is applied. If the physiotherapist does not apply over-pressure, the information she records is likely to be incorrect.

> A **joint's** movements can **never** be classed as normal unless *firm* over-pressure can be applied painlessly.

· When movement causes pain, measurement of the range should be based on that given in the booklet *Joint Motion. Method of Measuring and Recording*[1]. The method of examining these active movements will not be discussed here as reference to the booklet, which has been widely accepted for the benefit of universal standards, can be made separately. It is important to point out, however, that with some joints, if the movement is assessed first in the standing position and then in the supine position, different measurements will be recorded. This is more obvious in weight-bearing joints but it also applies to the shoulder joint where gravity assists flexion in the supine position but resists it in the standing position.

It is important that the person examining the patient's joint movements should take into account simultaneously both pain and range. When recording examination findings the physiotherapist should not record the range of movement which a joint may lack without also recording the site, type and degree of the patient's pain felt with that test movement. Similarly, she should not record any findings in relation to the patient's pain with movement unless it is also related to the range at which or through which the pain is felt.

> During examination and assessment **pain** should **never** be considered without relation to **range** nor **range** without relation to **pain**.

The effect of compression on weight-bearing joints while in the standing position can be an important consideration, being introduced into the examination of active movement to elicit joint pain. A common example is a patient with minor knee symptoms who may have a full painless range of active knee movements when tested in a supine position but when asked to stand and squat fully, finds flexion is very painful.

During examination, if a joint sign comparable to the patient's symptoms cannot be found, the patient may be able to recall the

---

[1] *Joint Motion. Method of Measuring and Recording* (1976). 7th Reprint. American Academy of Orthopaedic Surgeons

exact movement which caused his injury. Gentle repetition of this movement, simulating the condition under which the injury occurred, should be used as a test. However, not all joint pain has a traumatic origin and details of trauma cannot always be recalled.

If the physiological movements are tested and no positive signs are found, the joint involved should be subjected to strongly resisted active movements under load. Performing the movements against gravity may be sufficient load to provide joint signs but if this is not so then increased resistance must be included in the test movement.

STATIC TESTS

Muscles which lie under the area of the patient's pain should be tested strongly isometrically to see if the pain can be thus reproduced. At the same time, notice should be taken of muscle power.

OTHER JOINTS IN 'PLAN'

Routine examination must always include quick tests of the joints above and below the painful one so that, hopefully, they can be excluded from the clinical examination; if found to be limited or painful then they will have to be examined in detail. The relevant area of the spine should also be examined.

PASSIVE MOVEMENTS

One of the main functions of examination by passive movement is to find a movement or movements with signs (pain, resistance or spasm) which can be compared to the patient's symptoms. If more than one such movement is found, their respective signs are compared. For example, during the examination of a man who has pain encompassing the right shoulder region all movements of the glenohumeral and acromioclavicular joints are tested passively to determine the extent and nature of limitation of the movements and the pain which may be present in each direction. The important examination findings are those movements which produce pain comparable to the symptoms, while the movements which produce a small amount of pain become less important. The movements are recorded in order of severity and any loss of range in each of these directions is also noted.

Passive movements can be broadly divided into two groups. The first is the group of active movements which can also be performed passively, i.e. passive physiological movements. In the second group movements are not under voluntary control and can only be produced passively, i.e. passive accessory movements. For example, shoulder flexion is a physiological movement whereas movement of the head of the humerus up and down in the glenoid cavity is an accessory movement. Although the gross range of both passive and active physiological movements is similar, the joint-surface relationships during their movements are not necessarily so. For example, as soon as muscles contract to produce active movements the joint surfaces are compressed. During passive movements there is no compression unless the examiner deliberately applies it. Another difference relates to the gliding of the joint surfaces which occurs during movement. This is best seen in the glenohumeral joint. The glenoid fossa is shaped to allow an upward and downward movement of the head of the humerus. While the arm hangs by the side of the body, the head of the humerus occupies the upper part of the glenoid cavity, and as the arms are raised above the head the muscular action moves the head of the humerus downwards in the glenoid cavity. When the arm is raised actively, the head of the humerus, at any one position in the range, always occupies a constant position in the glenoid cavity. If, however, the same position in the range is maintained passively, the head of the humerus can be moved into various positions in the glenoid cavity. Thus, it is possible to perform passive accessory movements during passive physiological movements.

The need to use compression to elicit joint signs was discussed in relation to testing active movements. When passive movement tests do not elicit pain they should be repeated while compression is applied. This is not so easily managed in joints such as the hip and shoulder, but in other joints such as the hand and foot where compression is most commonly needed in examination, it is fortunately easier to apply.

The first movements to be tested passively should be those which have been tested actively. These tests are repetitious of the active movements given in the booklet *Joint Motion. Method of Measuring and Recording*[1] performed as passive movements, and as such will not be described here. However, there are test movements not included in the above booklet which form an important part of examination

---

[1] *Joint Motion. Method of Measuring and Recording* (1976). 7th Reprint. American Academy of Orthopaedic Surgeons

when the routine test movements do not give conclusive answers. These will be described in detail in the chapters relating to each joint.

As relaxation is essential for effective testing of passive movements the tests should be performed with the patient in a reclining position. It is the position of choice even when a joint such as the wrist is being examined.

Firstly the patient should be asked if he feels any pain, and if he does, its site should be determined. The joint should then be moved through the range to the position where pain is first felt and this position should be noted. Then the joint should be moved further, the physiotherapist watching the patient carefully to assess the degree of pain being experienced. Unless the pain becomes excessive, the joint should be moved to the limit of the range. The available range together with any change in the site or degree of pain should be recorded. The nature of the limitation, whether it be muscle spasm or stiffness, should also be noted. This assessment should be made for each direction of movement which has been performed actively so that a comparison between the active and passive movements can be made. A discrepancy between a range of movement performed passively and actively may be due to loss of muscle power or an inability to move further because of pain. This text is concerned solely with joint-pain problems and excludes those disturbances of movement which are due to loss of muscle power or function and have a neurological origin.

ACCESSORY MOVEMENTS

Measurement of passive physiological movements is generally accepted as routine examination but it should be realized that the range of passive accessory movements can and must also be assessed; these latter, performed in different directions, are very small and their assessment is therefore more difficult. However, if the joint is to be treated by passive movement their assessment is most important. If the accessory movements are limited and painful, the active movements cannot be normal. A loss of range in one accessory movement can explain why a particular physiological movement is restricted.

Accessory movement tests should be considered in two ways. The first relates to joints such as the glenohumeral joint and the knee joint where large movements take place in a single joint. In these instances accessory movements, produced by thumb or hand pressure against the head of the humerus or tibia respectively, can readily be assessed for pain and range. In joints such as the sternoclavicular joint or acromio-clavicular joint these accessory movement tests may be the only tests to give positive findings. For example, if the sternoclavicular joint is the source of minor symptoms, the active and passive shoulder girdle tests of flexion, depression, protraction, retraction and rotation may be painless, while accessory movements of the joint performed with thumb pressures reproduce the deep pain. The temporomandibular joint is another familiar example.

The second aspect relates to a movement comprising the movement of many joints working in harmony, as in the hand. When active and passive wrist flexion are painful often it is only with accessory movement tests of the intercarpal and carpometacarpal joints, by thumb pressures or gliding intermetacarpal movements, that the painful lesion can be localized to a particular joint.

It was pointed out earlier that passive accessory movements are possible at any stage of flexion of the arm (*see* page 19). This principle applies for every joint, even when many joints work together, as in the hand. To examine accessory movement in different positions of the joint-range may be the only method of finding joint signs comparable to the patient's symptoms. As finding such a movement is sometimes missed because of difficulty in testing and lack of perseverance, treatment by passive movement may not be successful. For example, a patient who intermittently experiences sharp pain somewhere deep in the radial side of his hand while pouring the tea from a teapot may have active and passive physiological movements which reveal very little. However, careful examination may reveal that the sharp pain can be reproduced by a postero-anterior gliding of the first metacarpal on the trapezium if the joint is put under compression. The important point is that pain with this test movement is comparable with the patient's symptoms. Testing accessory movements in different physiological joint positions is frequently essential to determine the most painful or most limited part of movement.

Many anomalies occur in the clinical situation which do not entirely agree with what is known anatomically and physiologically. Description of movement between the capitate and hamate provides a useful example of the comparison between the theoretical considerations of a joint movement and the clinical assessments.

Under normal pain-free circumstances it should be possible to hold the capitate anteriorly and posteriorly around the lateral border of one hand with the middle finger and thumb while at the same time holding the hamate between the fingers and thumb of the other hand around the medial border of the hand. With this grasp it is quite easy to slide both bones back and forth against each other and to produce and feel movement at the joint. If the movement is stretched at each extreme and the joint is normal then the movement and stretching will be painless.

If a patient has pain in his hand which is felt during various functional movements, accurate examination of the intercarpal area may indicate, for example, that the pain is arising from the joint between the capitate and hamate because some of the movements occurring at the joint, when performed passively, reproduce the pain. *Figure 2.1* represents diagrammatically the normal relationship of the capitate–hamate joint.

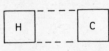

Figure 2.1. – Normal neutral position of the right hand under normal circumstances. View of the proximal surfaces of the hamate and capitate

Circumstances may exist where if the capitate is stabilized so that it does not move and the physiotherapist pushes the hamate anteriorly with her free hand, the patient's pain may be reproduced (*Figure 2.2a*). In theory the pain should also be reproduced if the same movement is stretched in the same direction but this time with the hamate being stabilized with one hand while the capitate is moved posteriorly with the other hand (*Figure 2.2b*). Clinically this is not always so even though theoretically the same movement is being produced by both methods. Importantly, the movement which reproduces the patient's

Figure 2.2. – (a) Capitate stabilized. Hamate moved anteriorly. (b) Hamate stabilized. Capitate moved posteriorly. Theoretically if one method of performing the movement is painful it is reasonable to expect that both ways of performing the same movement should be painful. However, clinically one can be painful (a) and the other pain free (b)

pain should be the movement used in treatment. The movements may be further investigated by comparing the movement described above firstly with the capitate and hamate distracted and secondly with them compressed.

The above description is related to only one movement of the joint between the capitate and hamate. Further examination of this joint is performed by producing postero-anterior pressures on the capitate, then on the hamate, and then on the joint line between the capitate and hamate (*Figure 2.3*). Each of these three postero-anteriorly directed pressures produces a different movement in the capitate–hamate joint and any one of them may reproduce the patient's pain, or one may be more dominant than the others.

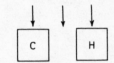

Figure 2.3. – Postero-anterior pressures on the capitate, the hamate, and the joint line

The joint movements produced by the postero-anterior pressures can be further varied by inclining them medially and laterally (*Figures 2.4a* and *b*), or cephalad and caudad (*Figure 2.5a* and *b*).

(a)   (b)

Figure 2.4. – Postero-anterior pressures directed (a) medially; (b) laterally

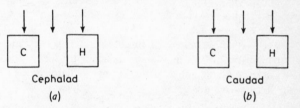

Cephalad   Caudad

(a)   (b)

Figure 2.5. – Postero-anterior pressures

All of these directions can be combined to test the various movements. For example, *Figure 2.6* shows one combination. It depicts movement between the capitate and hamate produced by a postero-anterior pressure combined with a medial inclination and a cephalad inclination. This pressure is applied at the joint line. The same direction of pressure could have been applied on the capitate or hamate.

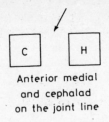

Anterior medial
and cephalad
on the joint line

Figure 2.6. – Postero-anterior pressure

Figures *2.3–2.6* all depict the left hand.

To test the joint still further, variations of pressure against each bone and the joint line should be done in the anteroposterior direction. Particular notice should be taken of

1. the position of bones in relation to each other (normal or abnormal);
2. the limitation of joint movement in any direction found with the examining palpation techniques;
3. the site and degree of pain produced by each of the movements: is it comparable with the patient's disorder?

The examination guides which technique should be used for treatment because the pressure techniques of examination can give such well defined detail.

Lastly, the clinical examination findings, bearing in mind the discussion above, will give information in relation to position, range of movement, and pain with movement. The manipulator is then able to decide whether treatment is going to be directed towards

1. restoring to normal the relationship between the capitate and hamate; or
2. increasing the range of movement between the capitate and hamate; or
3. making the available range pain free.

Thus, considerations related to the Principles of Treatment provide the manipulator with an exact knowledge of the movements and pain evident with the disorder and give a clear idea of the intention of the treatment technique.

As the passive tests used in examination are the same as those used in treatment, their description will be left until the joints are discussed individually. A general plan of the objective examination is given in Table 2.5.

Table 2.5
Objective Examination

Observation
    Watching for abnormal patterns of movement and willingness to move, deformity, swelling, inflammation etc.

Active movements
    Quick tests (active antigravity) of relevant joints
    Physiological movements (repeated, faster)
    Specific movements which aggravate
    The injuring movement
    Movements under load (antigravity or resisted)
    Resisted full-range if tendon sheaths involved

Static tests
    Test muscles under painful area for cause of pain and weakness

Other joints in 'plan'
    Joints above and below
    Relevant spinal area

Passive movements
    (These will be discussed in detail with each joint)
    Physiological movements
    Accessory movements with joint in a neutral position
    Accessory movements at limit of physiological range

Palpation
    Temperature, swelling, wasting, sensation, relevant tenderness and position of structures

Check case records and radiographs

HIGHLIGHT MAIN FINDINGS WITH ASTERISKS

After treatment
    Instruction regarding activities, rest, exercises and pain

With each test movement, assessment is made of the range of movement relative to the pain felt in each direction. From this information comparisons can be made between each direction of the joint's movements. However, range and pain alone do not give sufficient information to guide the manner in which the joint will be moved passively in treatment. Adequate detail is required in order to appreciate the relative position in the range of the onset of the pain and the onset of resistance, the type of resistance, the rate of increase in strength of each of these factors (that is, their behaviour during movement) and the relationship between these behaviours.

Some readers may consider this extent of detail unnecessary, but it should be realized that all experienced manipulators have this appreciation of joint signs and they modify their handling of a joint in accordance with small changes in the signs which occur during treatment. The finer the appreciation of detail, the better is the handling of the joint.

Teaching this perception in clinical terms to newcomers is exceedingly difficult. Not every patient is suitable demonstration material, and even when a suitable patient is available it is not possible, in the best interests of the patient, for all students to handle the joint. In addition and importantly, a teacher cannot be sure that newcomers have, in fact, felt what they should feel. Nevertheless, there will never be first-class handling and assessment of joint conditions unless the physiotherapist acquires a high degree of sensitivity to symptoms and signs in movements of the abnormal joint. New concepts of teaching this aspect of manual skill are needed, having, at least in part, a theoretical basis. If a theoretically based method can be used, students will come to handle joints more perceptively and learn far more from each experience which comes their way. Those students with little natural aptitude will be helped by having a theoretical basis for their work and a means of insight into what they should be able to feel.

> Geography would be incomprehensible without maps. They've reduced a tremendous muddle of facts into something you can read at a glance. Now I suspect economics is fundamentally no more difficult than geography except that it's about things in motion. If only somebody would invent a dynamic map.[1]

The Movement Diagram is a new concept which can be likened to such a map for economics and 'reduces a tremendous muddle of facts into something you can read at a glance.' The theory of the movement

---

[1]   Snow, C. P. *Strangers and Brothers* (1965), p. 67. Middx; Penguin Books Ltd

diagram is described in detail in Appendix I, and its practical compilation follows in Appendix II. It is the detail of Appendix II which the good manipulator must have, especially when related to palpation techniques of examination, as described on pages 20–24, and their use in treatment.

The complexity and subjectivity of the aspects of examination discussed here make them extremely difficult to learn. but unless they are learned, the handling of joints does not reach a high standard. Movement diagrams provide a method of gaining insight into the way these factors control, and are controlled by, the skilled use of movement both in examination and treatment.

3 Principles of Technique

To apply any technique of passive movement treatment the position adopted is governed by the following factors:

1. The patient must be completely relaxed if treatment is to be effective without placing unwarranted strain on the structures supporting the joint.
2. The patient must be comfortable and have complete confidence in the operator's grasp. The grip should not be tighter than that required to perform the movement and the position should make full use of the mechanical advantage of levers.
3. Wherever possible the operator should embrace the parts to be moved or stabilized. In accompaniment with this the operator should hold around the joint so as to feel the joint movement as the technique is performed.
4. The patient must feel confident that the joint will not be hurt by being moved further than he expects. The physiotherapist, therefore, must position herself carefully in such a way that she prevents the movement going beyond an established point.
5. The operator's position must be comfortable, easy to maintain and the most economical in which to carry out the treatment with minimum effort.
6. The operator's position must afford her complete control of the movement.

Before carrying out a technique, the direction and type of movement to be used is determined from the joint signs and the starting position adopted. The patient must be in a comfortable, fully supported position so that complete relaxation is possible and the physiotherapist must have complete control of the part to be moved. Whenever possible, part of the grasp must be around the joint so that the movement can be felt. During treatment minor changes may be needed, depending upon the 'feel' of the movement; smaller or larger amplitudes might be used or the movement performed earlier or later in the range than originally planned. These minor changes, which are made during small exploratory movements, also help to give the patient confidence in the physiotherapist's control. The technique is then performed for a planned period, and the patient's signs are then reassessed.

GRADES OF MOVEMENT

As will be evident from the previous chapter, any part of a range of movement may be used in treatment, and widely varying amplitudes may be chosen. It is both tedious and time-consuming to refer to a treatment movement as 'a large amplitude movement performed in the early part of the range' or 'a small amplitude movement performed firmly at the limit of the range.' To overcome this exigency, and to make the recording of treatment quicker and simpler, a system of grading movement is used. Although recording treatment will be discussed in detail later, it is necessary to introduce these grades of movement here because of their application to the treatment techniques in following chapters. Grades from I to IV are used to describe the treatment movements but like all similar gradings (for example rating of muscle power) the values overlap; that is there is also a place for plus and minus values. The grades of movement which are described below can be depicted in relation to a straight line representing a full range of movement (*Figure 3.1*).

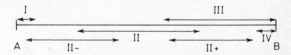

Figure 3.1. — Grades of movement. A = beginning of range of movement; B = end of normal average range of movement

Grade I: Small amplitude movement performed at the beginning of the range.

Grade II: Large amplitude movement performed within the range but not reaching the limit of the range. If the movement is performed near the beginning of the range it is expressed as II — and if it is taken deeply into the range, yet still not reaching the limit, it is expressed as II + (*Figure 3.1*).

Grade III: Large amplitude movement performed up to the limit of the range. This movement can also be expressed with plus and minus values. If the movement knocks vigorously at the limit of the range it is expressed as III + but if it nudges gently at the limit of the range it is expressed as III —.

Grade IV: Small amplitude movement performed at the limit of the range. This too can be expressed as IV + or IV — depending on its vigour as described for grade III.

If the normal range of joint movement is limited by the joint disorder grades III and IV are restricted to the new limit of the range, and grade II movements are restricted to smaller amplitudes (*Figure 3.2*).

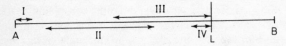

Figure 3.2. – Restricted grades of movement. A = beginning of range of movement; B = average anatomical limit; L = pathological limit of range

Similarly pain may arise from a hypermobile joint which is slightly stiffened. Such a situation alters the positions of grade III and IV movements as shown in *Figure 3.3*.

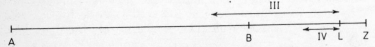

Figure 3.3. – Grades of movement in a hypermobile joint. A = beginning of range of movement; B = average anatomical limit; L = pathological limit of range; Z = a patient's limit of normal hypermobile range

The oscillatory treatment movements may be smooth and regular or performed with an irregular rhythm. When the treatment movement is carried into the painful range and the patient finds it difficult to relax, the treatment movement must be regular, it must be performed a little slower than usual and the rhythm must be even. The patient will then know exactly how his joint is to be moved and will find it easier to relax. Some patients have difficulty in relaxing completely even when pain is minimal. They periodically tense their muscles without realizing they do so. If large amplitude treatment movements are hindered by this tensing, movements of broken rhythm and changing amplitude should be employed in an attempt to trick the muscles. Sometimes the movements need to be performed almost as a flick. When a technique is initially used in treatment, it is commonly employed in an exploratory manner to determine the response of the joint. In this way the treatment movement is continually modified to meet the demands of the condition. The movements used will vary in depth, gradually moving in deeper and receding according to what is felt at different depths. Under other circumstances the treatment movement used is regular and rhythmical.

Many techniques are performed in positions similar to those used for examination; others have different positions for the operator. The physiotherapist tests many directions of movement during examination, each being performed only once or twice. This may indicate the use of one position. In treatment the movement is repeated many times in only one direction although the position may alter.

The gentler grades of movement sometimes require different starting positions from the stronger grades. The positions described are suitable for learning the various techniques but they may not suit all physiotherapists. Therefore, as the skill is learned and the feel of joint movement becomes instinctive, each physiotherapist should modify the positions to suit her own circumstances.

Of the many techniques described in the following text some are used commonly, others less commonly and some on a few occasions only. From a teaching point of view not all techniques must be taught in detail. If the principles and application of the important ones are understood this will be enough to ensure that the least important ones can be done when the need arises. Their presence in the text shows how techniques can be modified to suit unusual circumstances. The most commonly used techniques are marked with three asterisks (***), the less commonly used with two asterisks (**), and the techniques which are used least and need not be taught in detail at the undergraduate level with one asterisk (*).

Where applicable, techniques will be applied to the joints on the right side of the body. The patient will be referred to as 'him' and the physiotherapist as 'her' although the operator is depicted as male in the figures. The physiotherapist is called 'her' in order to emphasize the fact that brute strength is not essential to the use of manipulative treatment—rather, what is required are perceptive hands and an agile, methodical mind. Unless otherwise stated the patient will be lying supine for all techniques. Each joint will be described separately and more than one starting position may be given for one direction of movement.

4 Treatment:
Method and Assessment

The procedure for treating joint disorders by passive movement follows very definite lines. After examining the patient, the physiotherapist selects which technique she will use and decides what 'the intention of the technique' will be; that is, whether the technique will be aimed at relieving pain or stretching a stiff joint. To know this 'intention' is important because it must be taken into account when assessing the effect of each treatment technique.

The physiotherapist then positions the patient and performs the technique for a period varying between half-a-minute and one-and-a-half minutes. The length of time spent doing the technique depends upon the patient's pain and the likelihood of exacerbation from treatment. Longer techniques are reserved for the more chronic disorders.

Following this short period of treatment movement the patient is requested to stand and is asked if the symptoms have altered as a result of the technique. Following this subjective assessment the painfully restricted movements are reassessed so that the value of the treatment technique can be evaluated. Depending upon the subjective and objective assessments, the technique is repeated at the same strength, more gently, or more strongly. If the assessment indicates an unfavourable response, a different technique is used. If there are no changes it is wise to repeat the technique and if the second application does not improve the symptoms and signs, the technique should be discarded. A second technique is then selected and the same process of assessment is continued; that is, after the treatment technique is performed its effect is estimated by the patient's response, both subjectively and objectively.

The number of times and the number of techniques which are used at any one treatment session will be based upon the behaviour of the patient's pain. If the pain is severe then the amount of treatment movement has to be limited. On the other hand, if the condition is chronic in nature and the patient's pain is minimal, then additional mobilization can be carried out at a treatment session. The upper and lower limits of actual mobilizing times are 10 minutes and 20 seconds respectively. Most patients will require, at any single treatment session, three or four 1-minute applications of a single technique.

It may be difficult to know how much treatment to give on the first day, subsequent to the examination of joint movement. However, when the patient is seen the second time, the changes in his pain and the objective assessment of his movements, will clearly indicate how much treatment can be given at each treatment session.

ASSESSMENT

The next part of passive movement treatment, the part which makes this particular kind of treatment so informative, is 'Assessment'. The term 'Assessment' is used with two meanings.

1. The first meaning includes (a) interpreting the history of the patient's disorder, his symptoms and signs, so a diagnosis can be made; (b) determining the stage in the natural history of the disorder; and (c) the psychical effect the disorder is having on the patient, taking into account his ethnic background, his home and his job situation.
2. The second meaning refers to determining the effect the treatment has had by checking the patient's symptoms and signs after each application of every technique to determine the effect the treatment has had. This assessment is used to prove the value of the technique used at that particular stage of the disorder.

Of vital importance to the manipulative physiotherapist is knowledge of the behaviour of the patient's pain, of the stiffness and the muscle spasm, their inter-relationships and their relevancy to the disorder.

There are four times when Assessments are used:

1. *At the initial examination and treatment session*
2. *During a treatment session and also over a period of treatment*
3. *At the end of treatment*
4. *To assist in differential diagnosis*

ASSESSMENT AT THE INITIAL EXAMINATION

After the examination of a patient has been completed a doctor may or may not be certain of the diagnosis. It is not uncommon for a patient to have symptoms and signs indicating a musculoskeletal disorder. However, time and an atypical response to treatment may later lead to a diagnosis of more sinister origin. It is inconceivable therefore that a physiotherapist should treat unreferred patients. To do so would mean that the physiotherapist would undertake the responsibility for the diagnosis. Such practice is to be condemned. Physiotherapy, particularly passive movement treatment for the spine, should only be carried out under circumstances where there is the closest liaison between patient, physiotherapist and the referring doctor. This is without doubt in the patient's best interests.

ASSESSMENT RELATED TO DIAGNOSIS AT THE INITIAL EXAMINATION

Even though the referring doctor has examined and diagnosed the patient's condition before referral, the physiotherapist re-examines the patient at the initial interview. By bringing together all the examination findings, an assessment is made of the present stage of the disorder.

Even when the doctor has been able to make a diagnosis this does not give all the information the physiotherapist needs in order to treat by passive movement. The passive movement signs need to be examined in detail.

Diagnosis is a coadjutant factor linked with a patient's presenting history, symptoms and signs. In fact, an initial diagnosis may need to be changed when in retrospect it is seen how the patient's symptoms and signs alter with passive treatment.

Some doctors consider that a patient can have only one diagnosis. There are instances, however, when careful assessment and skilful planning of passive movement treatment will show that a patient having pain (say) from the base of the neck radiating to the shoulder and mid-upper arm may have two conditions. He may have a shoulder disorder causing the shoulder and arm pain coupled with a cervical joint disorder causing the neck and scapular pain. Examination of the joint signs for both the cervical spine and the glenohumeral joint should be accurately assessed at the initial examination. If joint signs are found both in the shoulder and in the appropriate cervical intervertebral joint, then ideally treatment should be applied to the cervical spine first. The joint signs in the spine may improve, resulting in the patient losing neck and scapular pain but retaining the shoulder and arm pain. Re-examination of the glenohumeral joint may reveal that the glenohumeral joint's signs have remained unchanged. Under these circumstances treatment should then be applied to this joint in an effort to clear its signs, so gaining an improvement in the shoulder and arm pain. There are many such examples of combined joint involvements to explain the different pain patterns which occur.

ASSESSMENT RELATED TO MOVEMENT AT THE INITIAL EXAMINATION

The manipulative physiotherapist bases most of her selection of techniques on the patient's history, symptoms and signs. As has already been said, this does not imply that diagnosis is unimportant. Changes of treatment techniques are guided by changes in the 'behaviour' of the pain and the 'behaviour' of the joint stiffness on testing movements. Behaviour of pain during joint movement is the most important aspect of examination and also the most important aspect to assess continually during treatment.

Examination of joint movements must be made with care to ensure that assessment by re-examination will be accurate.

As the first use of technique is gentle, any worsening of the signs by passive movement treatment will be minimal and not harmful. In fact the changed signs will be most informative.

There is yet another problem associated with assessment of a patient's movements and his pain. One movement, or a group of movements may be found to reproduce a particular part of the patient's symptoms while a different movement reproduces a second part of the patient's pain. Allied with this is the fact that it is *not uncommon* for a patient to have more than one kind of pain—either in the same area or in a closely linked area. The physiotherapist must be fully aware of these possibilities lest differences be missed during examination. For example, it is common for a patient to complain of two distinctly different kinds of headache, or of different pains in the hand or foot. The patient must be adequately questioned to determine the differences and each pain should be examined, treated and assessed independently.

The behaviour of joint stiffness should now be considered. In the normal person the movement of one joint surface on its companion is a friction-free movement. However, on examination of a patient's disordered joint, even though the range may be full, movement through the range may not be friction-free throughout. With experience it is possible to feel slight resistance to movement even though the range is full. This slight resistance is occasionally accompanied by crepitus, though this is by no means always the case. It is important that physiotherapists develop the skill of picking up this lack of friction-free smoothness.

When a joint is limited by stiffness, resistance may behave in either of two ways:

1. In the first part of the joint's movement slight restriction of the friction-free movement may be felt through a large part of the range and it only increases markedly in strength at the limit of the range; or

2. resistance may be felt in the range and the further the movement is carried into the range the stronger is the resistance, until it reaches the point where the physiotherapist is not prepared to stretch the joint further. In other words, the rate of increased strength of the resistance is proportional to the amount of the movement through range.

The physiotherapist must realize that these variations in joint stiffness can and do exist. Proficiency in assessment of their differences will only come with clinical experience.

At the initial examination it is behaviour of pain, of resistance, and of muscle spasm that form the basis for selecting treatment techniques. On rechecking (i.e. assessing) the original abnormal movements, it should be possible to interpret the value of a technique as applied to that particular joint, at that particular stage of the disorder. This is the whole purpose of assessment: *proving* the *value* of each treatment technique.

When recording the examination findings in the case notes, the important findings, which on reassessment will clearly and objectively reveal changes as a result of treatment, should be highlighted by marking them with an asterisk to facilitate reference back to them.

ASSESSMENT DURING TREATMENT

Assessment of changes in the symptoms and signs which occur as a result of treatment is made at the following times:

1. At the beginning of each treatment session.
2. During the carrying out of a treatment technique.
3. Between each treatment technique used during a treatment session.
4. As a retrospective assessment after a period of say five sessions.

ASSESSMENT AT THE BEGINNING OF EACH TREATMENT SESSION

This assessment needs to be carried out in a particular manner. The patient's interpretation of the effect of treatment at three times are very valuable. These times are:

(a) immediately following treatment;
(b) during the evening of the day of treatment; and
(c) on first getting out of bed the morning following treatment.

It is wrong however to ask the patient directly about his symptoms at these times. Questioning should be so planned that the physiotherapist can evoke spontaneous remarks which are then more informative.

When assessing at the beginning of a treatment session, the first question should be 'How have you been?' The answer will be valueless if the patient, interpreting the question as a general remark, answers 'Fine thanks, how are you?' The advantage of an initial, spontaneous, informative reply has been lost. However if the patient says, 'I can't believe it, I'm much better thank you,' then highly valuable information has been received.

If the first question produced a valueless answer, the next question should be, 'What do you feel was the effect of yesterday's treatment?' If the reply is 'Better' or 'Worse', further clarification is needed. In wishing to emphasize his present pain the patient may give the impression that he is worse, whereas on closer questioning, it may be shown that he was better after his treatment until he performed some activity whigh aggravated his pain. In these circumstances the treatment helped his disorder rather than made it worse. This kind of information may be gained through the following questions:

(a) 'In what way is the pain worse—is it more severe, sharper, changed to a throbbing pain, or has it increased in area, etc., etc.?' Then ask,
(b) 'When did it start to become worse?'
(c) 'What do you think made it worse?' 'Was it related to treatment or did you do something which may have aggravated it?'

The physiotherapist must be prepared to accept the possibility that she has performed a technique too strongly. If a patient comes in feeling cross, saying, 'What you did to me yesterday made me a lot worse', the beginner is going to feel very uncomfortable and disconcerted and perhaps not know how to handle the situation. She will find it easier to accept the blame if she can honestly reply 'Good! Not that I wanted to make you worse but it shows me exactly where I am going with the treatment', or 'If I can make it worse by too much or too heavy mobilizing then I should stand a good chance of being able to improve it.'

If the vital spontaneous information is not forthcoming it may be necessary to ask the direct questions:

(a) 'How did you feel when you left here after treatment compared with how you felt when you came in?'
(b) 'How did you feel for the rest of that day and that night?'
(c) 'How did you feel when you first got up the next morning?'

Should the answers still not give a clear assessment, the physiotherapist may need to ask, 'Have your symptoms altered at all as a result of treatment?' If the patient has to hesitate before answering, then it is fairly clear that the symptoms have not changed much, if they have changed at all.

If the patient reports feeling better from the treatment it is equally important ı ᵗ clarify what it is that has improved and in what way.

The abo ᵗe is the *subjective* assessment of the effect of the previous treatment. This is followed by the *objective* assessment which is achieved by retesting the previously abnormal movements and assessing the quality of any change resulting from treatment. Changes in these signs will, hopefully, agree with the findings of the subjective assessment, so that both sets of findings reinforce each other. The total assessment will then be more reliable.

ASSESSMENT DURING THE PERFORMING OF A TREATMENT TECHNIQUE

When carrying out a passive movement technique, the physiotherapist should first ascertain whether the patient has any pain while positioned for the technique.

The movement is then performed at a chosen grade and the patient is asked whether the technique is causing any alteration to the symptoms. This information is helpful from three points of view.

(a) The patient may have referred pain while positioned for treatment. As the treatment technique is performed this pain may gradually lessen and disappear, it may remain at the same level throughout, or it may worsen. Assessment during the performance of the technique will guide whether to continue with the technique, to perform it more gently, or whether a change of technique is indicated. For example, if in the early stages of treatment of a patient who has shoulder pain, performing the technique initially causes an increase of the pain, and this pain worsens as the technique is continued, then that technique should be discontinued. The physiotherapist should stand the patient and reassess the movement signs before going on to the next technique.

On the other hand, if the condition is chronic in nature it may be necessary to provoke some pain with treatment technique if treatment is to be successful. On reassessment it would be hoped that the provocation had brought about a definite improvement in the pain-free range of movement.

(b) The patient may have no pain while positioned prior to performing the technique. Then during performance he may feel pain. The physiotherapist may choose to continue with the same technique at the same grade and ask the patient three, four, five or six times during the performance whether the pain remains the same, improves or worsens. If pain increases she may then lessen the grade of the technique, or stop. However, she may do it more firmly if there is no change in the symptoms or if they improve.

(c) There is one other response which can be determined during treatment. It is a difficult assessment to make but it is useful to know, when performing a technique, whether the pain is provoked only at the limit of the oscillation. The easiest way to make this assessment is to ask the patient while performing the technique, *'Does–it–hurt–each–time–I–push?'* These words are said in rhythm with the strongest part of the treatment technique. The patient easily understands the question if it is put this way and has no hesitation in answering informatively.

These assessments should be noted on the treatment record as discussed in Chapter 10.

ASSESSMENT BETWEEN TECHNIQUES DURING EACH TREATMENT SESSION

The main points to be considered under this heading have already been covered in the section on 'Assessment at the beginning of each treatment session'.

Care must be taken, firstly in the manner of questioning and secondly in the accuracy of testing movement which forms the basis of comparison.

Having carried out a treatment technique at a chosen grade long enough to expect some change in the patient's symptoms and signs, the physiotherapist asks the patient to sit up (or stand up) for the assessment. She then asks, 'How does it feel now?' If there is no immediate spontaneous response, she asks 'Is there any change?' Again, pertinent questioning and accurate interpretation devoid of assumptions are important.

The patient's movements are then retested and a comparison made with those present before the treatment technique was used. When reassessing the movement signs the same sequence of movements must be used each time. The reason for this is that one movement which provokes pain may alter the pain felt with the next movement tested. It is inconsistent to test movements one time in standing, another sitting in a chair, and a third time with the patient sitting on a treatment couch without foot support.

It is hoped that the subjective and objective assessments will agree.

In principle, when a physiotherapist is in the learning stages of 'treatment by passive movement', the above assessments should be made following each use of every technique. As experience is gained she learns to expect a certain degree of improvement when particular techniques are applied to particular disorders. However when a patient has movements which are almost painless but stiff, she can assume that there will be little change during one treatment session though there may be considerable improvement over two treatment sessions. In these circumstances it would be unnecessary to assess after each technique but comparison of the symptoms and signs at the end of the second treatment session should be made with those at the beginning of the first treatment.

If the physiotherapist is able to judge that changes in symptoms and signs may be expected to take place quickly, she should assess them after each application of a technique and if the *rate* of change is not as much as hoped for, then a change in technique should be made. This procedure should be maintained throughout the treatment, changing from technique to technique to find the one, or ones, which produces the quickest and best improvement.

RETROSPECTIVE ASSESSMENT

Even when it is possible to make confidently an objective assessment that progress has been made, it is still of value to know how the patient feels he is progressing.

When questioned regarding his symptoms, a patient's answer may well be influenced by factors related to his work, his home problems, litigation, his ethnic group, his desire to please the physiotherapist, etc., etc. Therefore the physiotherapist should endeavour to draw accurate answers to her questions, and to assess their meaning. In the context of question and answer she must *never assume anything*.

At the beginning of treatment it is not uncommon for a patient to reply, day after day, that he is feeling much better. Then, when asked after say four treatments, 'How do you feel compared with before we started treatment?', he may say cautiously, and after a long period of thought, 'I'm sure it's a little better—at least it certainly isn't any worse.' Such retrospective assessment alerts the physiotherapist so that she does not fall into the trap of believing she is making as much daily progress as she might have thought she was.

It can be of help to ask the patient, 'What percentage of progress do you think you have made since we began treatment?' If the patient finds it difficult to use percentages he may answer by some other comparison which is equally useful. The physiotherapist should make her own percentage assessment before putting the question to him. If there is agreement between her judgement and his, then obviously communication and assessment are good.

Sometimes the subjective and objective assessments do not agree. For example, a patient's pleasure at improvement in his symptoms may not be equally reflected by improvement in his signs. The converse can also occur. However, these are exceptions to the general rule and at a later stage of treatment, judgements may agree,

Even when a patient has clear objective signs on which assessments can be made, it is still important to find out how the patient considers he is progressing. It is poor policy to continue treatment time after time without making this 'retrospective assessment'. It is too easy to continue treatment unnecessarily, leading to perpetuating the joint disorder.

ASSESSMENT AT THE END OF TREATMENT

Assessment at the end of treatment is similar in many ways to the retrospective assessment discussed above. However, two aspects of the pathology should be taken into account when deciding whether or not treatment should be continued. The first of these is the stage of the pathology causing the joint symptoms and the second is related to 'what is normal in the way of pain and range of movement for the patient'. In other words, the goal of treatment may have to be a compromise rather than a 'cure'.

PATHOLOGY

When it is possible to be sure of the diagnosis then it is also possible to know what treatment can hope to achieve and whether recurrence of symptoms is likely.

An example of assessment related to pathology is worthy of consideration. A patient is referred by his doctor for treatment with a diagnosis of symptoms arising from a low grade osteoarthritis. The doctor appreciates that to regain a full painless range of joint movement is impossible but he believes that treatment will improve range .and lessen pain. The question is, when does one discontinue treatment?

In the early stages of passive movement treatment for such a patient a gratifying improvement in range and pain can be hoped for. Later, a stage during treatment will be reached when the patient's symptoms have improved but have now reached a static stage. It is probably difficult to be sure whether the range of movement is improving. The physiotherapist should be aware that a stage can be reached when, in fact, the mobilizing is perpetuating the complaint. At this point the patient can be asked the direct question, 'Do you feel you have continued to improve over the last three or four treatments at the same rate as when we began?' If the answer is 'No', then the concentrated treatment should be discontinued for a period of approximately two weeks, after which the patient's signs and symptoms should be reassessed.

On this reassessment:

(a) if the symptoms have improved, then the patient should be left for a further two or three weeks and reassessed again. If there is additional improvement, the patient can be discharged on the assumption that the symptoms will continue to improve without treatment.

(b) if the symptoms and signs have remained the same, the patient should be given four or five more treatments and then taken off treatment again for two weeks. At the end of this period it will be possible to determine whether the extra treatment resulted in any improvement or not, and therefore whether a further few treatments should be administered.

This pattern of 'treatment–break–assessment–treatment' is very useful but it must be very accurately assessed if it is to be used constructively.

It may be of interest to mention here that when these patients have recurrences, and they always do have recurrences, usually:

(a) they seek treatment at an earlier stage of the exacerbation;
(b) they respond more readily to treatment;

(c) they have progressively longer periods without exacerbation; and
(d) many of their exacerbations recover quite quickly without treatment.

'NORMALITY'

The second consideration is, 'What is normal in the way of pain and movement for this patient?'

People have widely differing norms. Many people 'live with' a certain amount of pain and stiffness. This can be present in any synovial joint and its supportive structures. These people consider their state to be normal. Other people have slightly stiff joints yet have no pain. Some people have painless hypermobile joints.

Realization of these possibilities coupled with careful assessment of treatment helps to put the patient's symptoms and signs, at the end of a period of treatment, in their proper perspective. If the physiotherapist decides to discontinue treatment, believing that she has reached the patient's norm, she should explain her reasons for doing so.

ASSESSMENT ASSISTING IN DIFFERENTIAL DIAGNOSIS

At the initial examination of a patient the doctor may not be able to make a definitive diagnosis. If the problem is a musculoskeletal disorder then under some circumstances passive movement treatment can be applied in such a way as to assist in making the diagnosis. For example, a patient may have shoulder pain. On examination joint signs can be found in both the neck and the shoulder. The actual cause of the pain may be in doubt. If the physiotherapist treats the cervical area first and improves its signs without any improvement in the shoulder then the neck is not the cause of the shoulder pain. However, if the shoulder symptoms and signs improve with the neck treatment then the neck was probably the source of the shoulder symptoms and signs. There are many examples similar to this which can be cited.

IN CONCLUSION

Just as there are communication difficulties in normal conversation between two people arising from misinterpretation of the meanings of things said, so there are difficulties in assessing a patient's subjective response to treatment. Because of these difficulties the physiotherapist should be *most* careful in questioning to assess any variations in the patient's symptoms.

None of the patient's feelings about his pain should ever be assumed. For example, if a patient is asked to raise his arm above his head, and as he does so he says 'Ouch!', the physiotherapist should immediately follow up with 'Did that hurt?' Patient—'Yes.' Physiotherapist—'Where did it hurt?', etc. Don't assume you know where it hurts.

As the examination continues and the patient repeatedly feels pain with each movement, it can be irritating to him to be continually asked 'Where did it hurt?' Under these circumstances, if the patient cringes during test movements, the physiotherapist can ask, 'In the same spot?' This avoids reiteration while still getting the correct message. Assume nothing. If the pain alters in its area he will say where it is, even if he is only asked 'In the same spot?' It is this close communication which assists assessment and thereby makes the treatment specific and more effective.

Although some will consider all of this is too time-consuming to be of value, successful treatment compels this degree of accuracy; it is essential if the physiotherapist is to remain in control of the treatment situation. Given practice and experience, it is not a lengthy procedure and it is very rewarding to both patient and physiotherapist.

5 Treatment:
Application of Techniques

Whenever passive movement is used in the treatment of joint disorders, the techniques applied are guided by both the diagnosis and the manner in which the joint and its inert supportive structures are affected. Diagnosis can directly influence the treatment technique in two different ways. Firstly, the diagnosis (such as that of rheumatoid arthritis) may indicate that structures supporting the joint will be weak; this will mean that the techniques must be performed gently. Secondly, a diagnosis of torn meniscus or loose body in a joint will mean that special techniques are required. However, there are very many times when an exact diagnosis cannot be given other than to state that the disorder is musculoskeletal and that it should respond to treatment by passive movement. Under these circumstances, the techniques used will be guided by the abnormalities of the joint movements.

The physical joint signs found on examination of an abnormal synovial joint and its supportive structures consist of pain, at rest or with movement, stiffness due to contracted structures or adhesions, and muscle spasm. These can be present separately or in any number of combinations. The following are the main situations which may pertain.

1. The joint may remain painful even when it is rested in a neutral position midway between all of the joint's possible ranges of movement.
2. A very important variation of the above situation is that the patient may say his joint is constantly painful yet if his joint is rested in a neutral position the pain will completely go. Although

it may not require much movement from this neutral position to become painful the important point is that it can be positioned to relieve the pain. The difference is that the pain which can be relieved may be caused by a mechanical focus whereas the example in No. 1 is more likely to be due to some active inflammatory condition.

3. A joint may be painless when at rest and only become painful on movement. There are many variations of the amount and type of pain felt on movement. The joint may give a sudden sharp pain on certain movements but as soon as the movement is stopped, pain immediately goes. At the opposite end of the scale, the joint may be very painful on movement and when the movement is stopped the pain may continue as an ache of varying intensity lasting varying lengths of time.

4. A joint may be painful at rest but if it is moved by the physiotherapist the pain increases rapidly in intensity to the extent where the physiotherapist is not prepared to move the joint further. The amount of limitation of movement due to pain may be very great and this prevents the physiotherapist from knowing whether there is any physical resistance present. She also cannot know whether there would be any muscle spasm if the joint were moved further. In other words it is not possible, because of the intensity of the pain with movement, to know what other physical factors may be present in the joint movement into the range.

5. The patient may have a painless joint which prevents normal activities because the joint is stiff. When the joint is stretched it may feel tight, and perhaps even a little painful, but the main complaint is one of stiffness rather than pain. This patient goes to his doctor because he cannot tuck his shirt into the back of his trousers or comb his hair but not because of pain.

6. The largest number of patients with musculoskeletal problems whom the doctor refers for physiotherapy are those whose joint is found to be both stiff and painful. These patients are the most challenging to treat. They require the physiotherapist to be precise in discerning the behaviour of the pain and the stiffness and to determine their inter-relationships. She must determine whether the behaviours of pain and resistance are associated with each other or not, either in part or in full. In making this interpretation it is necessary for the physiotherapist to know the diagnosis and understand the pathology. With this large group of patients the physiotherapist must build up a concept of the rate of anticipated change which can be affected

by manipulative physiotherapy. These skills can only be developed through precise examination of passive movements combined with continual assessment of changes which can be effected by different techniques.

7. A joint can be painless because of protection afforded by muscle spasm. The protective mechanisms in man are complex and wonderful. It is possible for the degree of muscle spasm to be such that it comes into play before movement becomes painful. It can also come into play as a more obvious protection for the joint because the joint movement becomes quite painful before the spasm appears.

There are two other kinds of muscle spasm which need not concern us in this text but should be mentioned. The first is a neurological muscle spasm caused by an upper motor neurone lesion and the second is the muscle contraction produced voluntarily by the patient to prevent movement.

Having described the components of joint disorders which can be determined during physical examination, an outline of the way passive movement treatment can be applied to the abnormal findings must be discussed. The treatment movements can be used in one of the following ways.

1. To direct the treatment to relieve the pain.
2. To direct the treatment so as to improve the painless stiff joint which does not have a functional range.
3. To treat the resistance present in the joint disorder while also being careful to avoid any exacerbation of the pain.
4. To reposition torn structures or loose bodies within a joint such that the joint can move painlessly through a full range allowing normal functional activities.

TREATMENT OF JOINT PAIN

Following examination of the patient's joint movements it may be determined that it is pain which is preventing an otherwise full range of joint movement. Special techniques performed in a special sequence can be used to treat this pain.

In another instance the examination may reveal that there is some joint stiffness but it is the pain rather than stiffness which concerns the patient most. Under these circumstances the pain should be treated first.

When both pain and stiffness are present it is wise to see firstly if treatment of pain can effect improvement. It is possible that the stiffness may disappear as improvement is achieved by treating and relieving the pain. Also, directing the treatment to the pain first will avoid unnecessarily strong treatment which may increase the patient's pain.

When pain is to be treated the following is the routine to be adopted. As the physiotherapist gains experience she may be able to take short cuts hoping for a quicker improvement.

The special type of passive mobilization used to treat pain makes use of the joint's accessory movements while the joint is supported in a neutral position. At a later stage the physiological movements are performed through a large amplitude. All of these movements are initially performed short of producing any discomfort or pain in the joint. As the condition improves they may be used into a controlled degree of pain. The accessory movements in a neutral position are chosen for those patients whose active antigravity movements are painful or uncomfortable in approximately the first 60 per cent of the joint's normal range. The change from accessory movements to physiological movements is made when the joint's pain-free range of movement has improved so that pain or discomfort is only felt in the last 40 per cent of its total range.

Assuming that the special passive movement techniques produce the desired improvement in range, progressive stages of the techniques are applied. If we take the example of a patient who has a glenohumeral range of approximately 15 to 20 per cent of (say) flexion before discomfort is felt then the steps are followed in this order:

1.   The joint is placed (if necessary by using pillows, etc.) in a pain-free position in approximately the middle of all the joint's ranges. The technique used is postero-anterior accessory movement, and while this is being performed very gently the physiotherapist should repeatedly ask the patient if he feels any discomfort. If he does, the oscillatory movement should be performed further back in the range and the question asked again. If there is still some discomfort during the technique then a much smaller amplitude should be used and it may be necessary to use a very gentle degree of distraction of the joint surfaces while performing the technique. It is essential at the first treatment that the patient should not feel any movement nor anything resembling discomfort during treatment. An example of the technique is shown in *Figure 6.23* (page 92).

2.   If the careful assessment at the second treatment session shows that there has been some lessening of pain and some small

improvement in the pain-free range of movement then the technique described above can be repeated. The physiotherapist must be prepared to proceed slowly; but as soon as it is advisable, as indicated by the improvement shown on assessment, the amplitude of the accessory treatment should be made larger and may also move into part of the range which is painful. On reassessment, if the pain-free active range improves and pain lessens then the accessory movement can be made larger and larger moving further and further into the range even though it is a little painful, until a stage is reached when full amplitude Grade III movements can be performed.

3. A stage will be reached when Grade III+ accessory movements can be performed with minimal discomfort and at this stage the patient's active pain-free range should have improved in range to 60 per cent. The treatment movement can now be changed from an accessory movement to a suitable physiological movement performed very gently and carefully as a grade II− movement and done in such a way as to avoid pain. The amplitude should be as large as possible, but initially it must be a pain-free movement. An example of the technique which may be used is shown in *Figure 6.4b* (page 70).

4. As the pain-free range improves still further, the movement can be moved further into the range and may be taken into a controlled degree of discomfort.

5. Gradually, the amplitude and vigour of the movement can be increased until a strong Grade III+ movement can be performed without pain (*Figure 6.5a* and *b,* page 71). When this stage is achieved the patient will be symptom free.

6. The method described is a standard routine which may be used for any joint when treating pain. However, it must be pointed out that the change-over from the vigorous accessory movements in a neutral position to the physiological large amplitude movement short of pain is not a clearly defined point. If the physiotherapist is in doubt as to whether to change over or not, it is usually wise to repeat the accessory movements for another two sessions and to make them as vigorous as possible. Then the change to physiological movements can be made but the initial application of these should be performed cautiously. On reassessment, if the joint has become more painful or the active range has worsened, the physiotherapist should revert to the accessory movement for a further two or three treatments. Then if the change to physiological movement is again made it should be a successful transition.

The above description has been related to joints which have no stiffness or muscle spasm. However, as has been mentioned earlier, the largest group of patients referred for treatment are patients who have both pain and stiffness. If the physiotherapist is new to the use of passive movement techniques then it would be wise for her to treat pain first before trying to increase the range of movement limited by the stiffness. If this procedure is followed, the method used for treating pain is exactly the same as that described above. It is possible that by treating pain, the active range will improve as the pain recedes. However, when the stiffness is quite marked, the treatment of pain will only effect a small degree of improvement and will quickly reach a stage when progress, as determined by assessment, ceases. When this occurs, the treatment of pain should be discontinued and treatment of stiffness instituted.

TREATMENT OF JOINT STIFFNESS

When painless stiffness restricts a patient's functional activity, the method of treatment is as follows:

1. One of the stiff, functionally limited physiological movements is chosen and the physiotherapist takes the joint to the limit of this range. At this point small amplitude oscillatory movements are applied for approximately two minutes, attempting to increase the physiological range.
2. Then, while holding the joint at the limit of this range the physiotherapist performs the accessory movements which are available at this position. These accessory movements are small amplitude, strong stretching oscillatory movements (*see* example page 329 and *Figure 9.12*, page 328).
3. The physiotherapist now repeats the movements performed in No. 1 above and then follows with those described in No. 2. This alternating between physiological and accessory movements is repeated three or four times at the initial treatment session. Assessment of progress is made during each treatment session and from treatment to treatment.
4. If the technique described above creates any soreness, this can be readily relieved by performing the physiological movement used for stretching but the movement would now be performed as a large amplitude movement slightly short of the stretching range so that little or no pain is felt by the patient. If treatment

soreness is minor then this grade III– technique would not need to be performed for very long. The converse also applies.

5. Usually, as the chosen physiological treatment movement improves in range, the other movements of which the joint is capable also improve. When this is so, only one physiological movement needs treating. However, an all-round gain is not always the case and it is sometimes necessary to change to a different physiological movement. The same routine of stretching the physiological movement and the accessory movements at the limit of the physiological range is performed.

6. When the patient's joint is markedly limited in range, more than one physiological movement and its accompanying accessory movements may be used. Where possible, opposite movements in sequence should be avoided. Treatment may be more effective if more emphasis is placed on the physiological movements even to the extent of omitting the accessory movements.

7. The physiotherapist may feel that the joint should be stretched more strongly in an endeavour to break whatever tight structures are restricting range. However, this should not be done unless the referring doctor agrees that it is necessary, and the patient must be fully informed. The technique is described on pages 114–116.

TREATMENT OF PAINFUL STIFF JOINTS

As has been mentioned before, the majority of musculoskeletal patients referred to physiotherapists fit this category. The physiotherapist first needs to determine whether the pain or the stiffness is the dominant problem. If she is in any doubt it is advisable to treat the pain first. This should follow the lines already described. If treating the pain produces no improvement, or if it has only limited success and the range of active movement ceases to improve, the physiotherapist must change her techniques so that her intention is to treat the stiffness. While treating stiffness with techniques similar to those described above for the painless stiff joint, if the patient feels pain (as he most certainly will) then the physiotherapist must appreciate its extent and its site so that she is alert to what she is subjecting the patient.

Treatment for a stiff painful joint is an important field for the manipulative physiotherapist. If firm treatment is done too strongly or at the wrong time, it will be unsuccessful and will cause unnecessary pain and will bring the treatment into disrepute. Nevertheless, it is a most important part of manipulation because it can be so dramatically effective when performed accurately.

The following is the routine which should be followed.

1. The initial treatment should be to determine what happens to the joint symptoms and signs when pain alone is treated. Over a period of one or two treatments it is possible to determine the behaviour of the pain and so know how it may limit any stretching-type techniques which may be used later.

2. The examination of the patient's joint should reveal the behaviour of the pain, the most restricted movements, and the pain felt when these movements are stretched. The painfully stiff movements should be correlated with the patient's loss of function and it should be determined whether it is the pain or the stiffness which limits the function. The direction of movement selected as the treatment movement should be the one directly associated with the loss of function; it will be the one which has 'comparable signs' as described in the chapter on 'Examination'.

3. When the comparable movement is used as the treatment movement, and where the intention is to stretch stiffness, a gentle grade IV movement should be applied, the physiotherapist being alert to changes in the patient's symptoms during the technique. This first treatment should be firm but not excessively painful though it must reproduce a degree of the patient's symptoms. If pain is only reproduced with firm pressure, then it is firm pressure which must be applied. The more easily the pain is reproduced the shorter should be the treatment time and the gentler the technique. If the joint can be stretched strongly with only slight pain then three or more separate stretches, each lasting one to two minutes, should be used. The reaction from treatment can be assessed the following day and this will guide the extent of further treatment.

4. If the patient has more than one site of pain arising from different joints or different areas from one joint, each should be treated separately. This situation frequently exists in the hand and foot.

5. As progress becomes more evident it is possible to treat the faulty joint by more than one movement and stronger grade IV movements may be used. How much is performed at a particular treatment session will be determined by the pain-reaction to treatment.

6. As was referred to in the section on 'Treatment of joint stiffness' treatment soreness can be readily relieved by using large amplitude movements in the painful direction but short of

pain. When stretching joints which are already painful these large amplitude comfortable movements are an essential part of treatment. Primarily they should be performed in the same direction as the stretching technique but other physiological directions may also be used.

7. When treatment of resistance does not produce an adequate rate of improvement, the next step is to consider manipulation. The method used is described on pages 114–116.

TREATMENT OF PAIN AND MUSCLE SPASM

The type of muscle spasm referred to in this section is that which occurs at the limit of the available range, is very strong, and occupies only a small part of the range.

1. As was mentioned in relation to the treatment of the stiff painful joint, it is wise to begin by treating pain and assessing its effect. Such treatment will give a good indication of the behaviour of the patient's pain and will also show the degree of irritability of the joint disorder. However, when such spasm is the most dominant sign which can be found on examination of the joint's movement, treatment of pain is unlikely to help.

2. The next step is to move the joint through a physiological range up to the point where spasm starts and there perform very small amplitude grade IV movements. These small passive movements can be used in conjunction with active relaxation techniques. If the range of movement does not improve and if the spasm shows no sign of relaxing it may be necessary to consider manipulation under anaesthesia. However, some orthopaedic surgeons prefer the manipulation to be carried out on the conscious patient because the patient can then provide the manipulator with instant information to direct the kind of technique used. However, other factors related to the patient's personality may sway the judgement in favour of the manipulation being performed under anaesthesia.

3. *Manipulation of the conscious patient.* When the physiotherapist has used further grade IV techniques, coaxing and stretching into muscle spasm or stiffness, she should balance how strongly she needs to push to increase range, against the degree of pain the patient experiences. Then, after consultation with the referring doctor if manipulation is indicated, one of two kinds of technique can be used.

(a) The first variety is applicable to small joints such as those in the hand and foot. Here, range is limited by stiffness not by muscle spasm. The technique is performed as a sudden very small amplitude thrust in the same position and direction as the stretching technique which reproduced the patient's pain. The pressure should be taken up first as a grade IV movement then increased to a grade IV+ and finally, superimposed on this pressure, the thrust is performed.

(b) When manipulation of larger joints is contemplated the technique is usually quite different. Here the joint may be protected by some degree of muscle spasm. The manipulation, rather than being a sudden thrust, is a controlled steady stretching technique. The patient must be positioned so that he is unable to move, in order that the physiotherapist can feel, in detail, what is happening at the joint during the stretching. A very close watch must be kept on the patient's hands and eyes as a means of assessing the amount of pain he feels during the technique. Once any tearing is felt the physiotherapist needs immediately to decide whether she is going to push right through the tear or whether she is going to ease her pressure, believing she will be able to have another stretch at a later date. The decision to go on or ease off is guided by the amount of pain being felt by the patient (that is whether the patient is likely to accept further stretching) and the type of tear. If it feels to be one thick adhesion it is better to push through it as the result is likely to be a good one in that full range will be restored quickly. On the other hand, the tear may be a soft, weak rupturing extending through a greater range. When this feeling is present it is better to do little at one stretch (*see* pages 114–116).

Learning the skill of this kind of manipulation can only be achieved under close supervision. The instructor, having selected the patient, should perform the manipulation with the novice's hands between her hands and the patient. This is necessary so that the juggling necessary to find the right direction for the stretch can be clearly appreciated. With this double-handed position, the novice can feel the slow controlled strength of the technique while also feeling and hearing the structures tear.

The physiotherapist should stabilize the patient with her body and arm, her hand supporting and feeling around the joint being manipulated, while at the same time the other hand stretches the joint (*see Figure 6.2*, page 67). Grade IV stretching is applied to the joint and the pressure is gradually increased until a point is reached when the spasm begins to release. It is usually at this stage that the abnormal structure releases and the range becomes full. The feel and sound of adhesions as they give way vary from a sharp snap which suddenly allows a full range movement, to a quiet slowly tearing sound.

TREATMENT RELATED TO PATHOLOGY

TO REPOSITION TORN STRUCTURES OR LOOSE BODIES IN JOINTS

The treatment used for the above purpose usually requires specific techniques. The joint must be distracted or opened to allow movement of the offending mechanical focus within the increased joint space. While the joint is opened on the painful side it should be moved back and forth in directions which will move the bones to which the loose piece is attached. By continuing the movement or varying the movements as dictated by progress or lack of progress the obstruction may be moved into a painless position, allowing the joint movement to become free.

RHEUMATOID ARTHRITIS

Passive movement techniques are never successful in relieving pain caused by an active rheumatoid arthritis. However, if the rheumatoid arthritis is not active and the patient complains of pain or aching of more recent origin, there may be a mechanical reason or minor recent trauma which is responsible for the pain. Under these circumstances gentle grade II type movements will be beneficial. However it will be necessary to carry out extremely gentle grade IV− techniques to relieve this pain. Firm techniques should never be used on joints exhibiting rheumatoid arthritic changes because the ligaments and tendons around the joint are structurally weakened by the rheumatoid disorder.

OSTEOARTHRITIS, OSTEOARTHROSIS AND TRAUMATIC ARTHRITIS

Passive movement has an extremely important part to play in the above disorders. The treatment technique will be directed towards either relieving pain by using large amplitude oscillatory movements, or towards increasing range when Grade IV— movements may be gradually increased to grade IV+ movements.

Pain resulting from osteoarthrotic joints or from long-standing traumatic arthritis can be very readily improved by large amplitude movements within range. When pain is severe, movements of large amplitude should be used but they should be performed painlessly as accessory or rotary movements in a neutral position. As pain recedes, large amplitude *physiological* movements should be used without provoking pain initially. As the condition continues to improve the large amplitude movements can be taken into pain and probably up to the end of the available range of movement.

HYPERMOBILITY

Hypermobility is not necessarily a pathological disorder. However, if it has a traumatic origin the hypermobility is pathological and perhaps it is then better to call it instability.

It is generally considered that a hypermobile joint should not be treated by passive movement. There are, however, two circumstances where such techniques can and should be used.

The first is if a hypermobile joint is painful. In this case, passive movement techniques can be used to relieve pain but they should not be strong stretching techniques which would increase the extent of hypermobility.

The second is when the patient requires increased mobility of a joint in a particular direction. The following example clarifies this point. A girl, aged 16 years, who had great promise as a ballerina, was referred for treatment because of pain she was experiencing in both knees following intensive ballet practice sessions. On examination she had no disability in her knees. On stretching both hips into the maximum abduction range while they were flexed to 90 degrees, the knee pains were reproduced. While she maintained the hips in this painful position, varying the position of her tibiofemoral joint made no difference to the pain felt in her knees. As would be expected, her range of hip movement in this direction was abnormally mobile. As this hypermobile range was not adequate for the work she was doing it was necessary to use strong passive stretching techniques to increase this range with the expectation that when she had the range she needed, the pain would go. This in fact has occurred and she is able to sit on the floor with her pelvis and trunk vertical while both legs are abducted fully to form a straight line in the coronal plane with both thighs on the floor; she has lost all of her knee pain.

RECENT FRACTURES

Injuries which result in fractures of the surgical neck of the humerus are usually severe enough to cause damage to ligaments and capsule, thus laying the basis for a stiff glenohumeral joint. Passive accessory movements of the glenohumeral joint in its neutral and supported position (*see Figure 6.23*, page 92) can play an extremely vital part in retaining maximum movement without any stress on the fracture. The importance of this early treatment cannot be over-emphasized; it is extremely important to realize that a good functional range can be retained without the fracture being subjected to stress (*see* pages 119–120).

Abduction is a very important glenohumeral movement. The movement can be performed as part of treatment in all fractures of the humerus if the full length of the humerus is supported throughout the movement with one arm while one or more fingers of the other hand assess movement between the head of the humerus and the acromion process.

This chapter has dealt with the techniques of passive movement as applicable to joint signs in a general way. In the chapters dealing with individual joints the techniques for that particular joint will be discussed more specifically. However the principles underlying the application of the technique are the same for all the moving parts.

Part II

JOINT TECHNIQUES AND MANAGEMENT

6 Shoulder Girdle

Before the techniques for each joint are discussed, special features peculiar to the joint will be described and related to examination and assessment. The full examination for each joint will not be dealt with in detail though a table will be given. Particular reference will be made to 'quick tests' and special tests'. The passive movement tests which form part of examination are also movements which can be used in treatment.

Examination of passive movements is very important and it is essential for the physiotherapist to know the feel of each joint's movements. This feel is important in two parts of a movement: the first is the friction-free feel through its full range and the second is the feel of the movement at the limit of the range.

QUICK TESTS

These are the first tests in the objective examination for the area concerned and consist in asking the patient to perform certain movements against gravity. They provide the physiotherapist with two important guides to examination.

1. They indicate the strength or gentleness required of the movements to determine the abnormalities.

2. They also show the patient's willingness to use the disordered joint. Any abnormal function provides the physiotherapist with a marker against which progress can be evaluated.

SPECIAL TESTS

Too often a joint is examined and classed as normal when if certain special passive movement tests were applied and compared with the normal side, minor abnormalities would not be missed. These special tests are usually movements made up of two physiological movements performed together, such as combining flexion and adduction of the hip, or a combination of a physiological and an accessory movement such as extension of the carpometacarpal joint of the thumb combined with a postero-anterior movement of the metacarpal on the trapezium.

The 'special tests' need only be used when the normal active physiological movements appear to be full range and painless. Before a joint can be classed as 'normal' overpressure should be able to be applied to these special test movements and the result found to be the same as for the sound joint on the other side of the body.

GLENOHUMERAL JOINT

The glenohumeral joint has large amplitudes of both physiological and accessory movements. These occur in a greater number of directions than in any other joint in the body. As a physiotherapist moves another person's arm passively through a physiological range, the accessory movements can be felt to be large also. This fact should be borne in mind when considering the selection of treatment techniques.

EXAMINATION

The full examination for a patient with general shoulder area pain will not be described. However a plan of the objective examination is given in Table 6.1. The symbols used in this and all subsequent examination tables are defined in Table 10.3 (page 336).

Table 6.1
Glenohumeral Joint: Objective Examination

Observation
   Watch for patient's willingness to move the arm when undressing—note abnormalities of appearance

Active movements
   Active quick tests (+cervical)

Table 6.1 (cont.)

Routinely
> F, Ab, behind back, HF
> Note range, pain, repeated, and behaviour (note scapular rhythm)

As applicable
> Speed of test movements
> Speed movements which aggravate
> The injuring movement
> Movements under load
> Thoracic outlet tests
> Muscle power

Static tests
> Rotator cuff
> Other muscles in 'plan'

Other joints in 'plan'
> Cervical spine
> Joints 'above and below'

Passive movements
Physiological movements
> *Routinely*
>> 1. F, $\circlearrowright$, $\circlearrowleft$, Ab, HF, HE, components of hand behind back; or
>>
>> 2. Quadrant and locking position
>> Note range, pain, resistance, spasm and behaviour

Accessory movements
> *As applicable*
> May be assessed at first session or as treatment progresses:
>> 1. By thumb pressures or arm leverage $\updownarrow$, $\uparrow$, ↢caud, ↢ or ↣
>>   (*a*) In different positions in the range
>>   (*b*) With addition of compression and/or distraction
>> 2. 1st rib
>> Note range, pain, resistance, spasm and behaviour

Palpation
> Temperature
> Swelling, wasting
> Altered sensation
> Relevant tenderness (capsule, tendons, bursa etc.)
> Position

Check case records and radiographs

HIGHLIGHT MAIN FINDINGS WITH ASTERISKS

After treatment
> 1. Warning of possible exacerbation
> 2. Request to report details
> 3. Instruction in 'joint care' if required

During the subjective examination, it is often useful when attempting to determine the site of pain to grasp around the head of the humerus so that the fingers on one side of the glenohumeral joint can press into the space between the humerus and the glenoid cavity towards the thumb pressing in on the opposite side of the joint. At the same time the physiotherapist can ask the question, 'Is the pain "in" [meaning deep within] here?' To emphasize the 'within' aspect of the question, the fingers and thumb gently rock the joint backwards and forwards. It may be necessary to support the acromioclavicular area with the other hand. The emphasis with which the patient is able to say 'Yes' or 'No' to the question has very real value.

QUICK TESTS

Among the many tests of the active movements, those of flexion and abduction should be done in a specific sequence to make the tests more accurate.

Flexion

1. The physiotherapist stands behind the patient. She asks him to lift both arms forward and above his head; she is careful not to touch him, so that he will not be influenced in his manner of lifting them. The movement will be a spontaneous one: he will raise his arm through its most comfortable range to the maximum height he can reach. While the patient is performing this movement the physiotherapist watches (a) the scapulothoracic rhythm; (b) the degree of abduction which he spontaneously uses during the flexion; (c) the manner of his movement throughout his range, that is, she assesses whether he has to move the arm slowly because of pain or is able to move quite quickly; and (d) the extent of the range.

2. Having noted all that can be seen in relation to the spontaneous flexion, the physiotherapist, while still standing behind the patient, then gently rests her hands on the lateral aspect of his elbows. She asks him to again raise his arms above his head but this time he keeps his arms closer together. She uses her hand position on his elbows to ensure he flexes in the sagittal plane. His range of flexion and behaviour of pain is then recorded.

Abduction

1. While still standing behind the patient she asks him to raise his arms sideways and above his head while she watches the spontaneous manner in which he performs the movement. She notes the degree of horizontal flexion, forward of the frontal plane, through which the patient moves his arm and notes when it begins and the manner in which it increases.

2. The patient is again asked to abduct his arms but this time the physiotherapist gently holds both arms back in the frontal plane. This countering of horizontal flexion will probably considerably limit the patient's range of abduction of the painful arm. This new range is noted and recorded.

Hand behind back

Another important functional test movement is to ask the patient to put his hand behind his back as high as he can reach. When he has reached this position the physiotherapist should then hold the patient's arm and endeavour to find out whether his inability to reach a full range is due to limited or painful glenohumeral extension, adduction or medial rotation. *Figure 6.13* (page 81) shows the test being applied to the patient in lying.

These tests provide valuable markers against which to assess the changes which treatment makes.

Rotator cuff

The muscles and tendons forming the rotator cuff can be quickly and easily assessed while the patient is standing for the preceding tests. As required, the tests can be performed more finely when the patient is supine.

SPECIAL TESTS

It is not uncommon for a patient with shoulder pain to be able to flex, abduct and place his hand behind his back in a manner exhibiting an apparent full range. Firm overpressure should then be applied to these movements.

If the three active quick tests are normal even when overpressure is applied, the physiotherapist should then test passively the 'quadrant' and the 'locking position', with the patient lying supine. Only if these tests are negative can the physiotherapist say the glenohumeral joint's movements are normal.

These two tests are unique in that they have not previously been recorded. They must be included in examination for they may be the only movements which indicate that the joint is not fully normal. These movements which will now be described can then be used as treatment movements to relieve a patient of his symptoms.

Locking position***

To find the locking position the patient lies supine and the physiotherapist abducts the patient's arm from alongside his trunk and endeavours to reach a position of full flexion.

She places the distal third of her near-side forearm under the medial border of the patient's scapula. Her thumb lies immediately adjacent to the vertebral column and she extends her fingers over the trapezius to prevent the patient's shoulder from shrugging. She holds his flexed elbow in her left hand, maintaining slight medial rotation and extension during abduction.

Provided the patient's upper arm is maintained in the frontal plane just posterior to the median frontal plane, the humerus will reach a position where it becomes locked. The humerus cannot be moved further towards the patient's head; neither can it be laterally rotated or moved forward from the frontal plane (*Figure 6.1*).

A patient whose symptoms are minimal or intermittent may appear to have a full painless range of active movement whereas if the locking

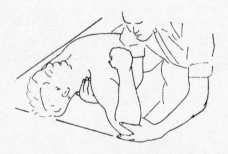

Figure 6.1. – Glenohumeral joint; locked

position is tested, it may be found to be abnormal and any attempt to push the glenohumeral joint into the locking position will reproduce pain. This same test movement should be applied to the normal shoulder to compare pain and range and so determine the extent of the disability. The locking position should always be examined when signs are minimal.

Quadrant***

To reach a fully flexed position from the locked position, the pressure maintaining abduction should be relaxed slightly to allow the arm to be moved anteriorly from the frontal plane. Lateral rotation can then take place as the abduction movement continues. This anterior and rotary movement takes place in a small arc of the abduction movement (this arc is the quadrant position) and the arm can then drop back behind the median frontal plane and continue its movement until the upper arm is alongside the patient's head (*Figure 6.2*).

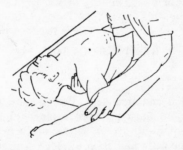

Figure 6.2. – Glenohumeral joint; quadrant

The quadrant is that position, approximately 30 degrees lateral to the fully flexed position, where the patient's upper arm has to move anteriorly from the 'locked' position. If the physiotherapist maintains pressure at the centre of the arc of the quadrant, pushing the patient's elbow towards the floor, the upper arm can then be rolled back and forth over the top of the quadrant. To do this successfully it is necessary to control the extent of medial and lateral rotation during the movement through the arc.

To examine the quadrant and locking positions the following procedure should be used.

1. The physiotherapist should put the patient's arm in the quadrant position and apply a reasonable degree of pressure, pushing the patient's elbow towards the floor. She should record the range in this position by observing two things:

   (*a*) the range of movement in the sagittal plane between the humerus and the anterolateral surface of the scapula; and
   (*b*) the extent of the prominence of the head of the humerus in the axilla.

2. While the patient's arm is oscillated anteroposteriorly in the quadrant position as a grade IV or IV+ the physiotherapist should take note of the site and degree of pain produced by the manoeuvre. The range and pain should then be compared with that present in the normal shoulder. As the positions are usually uncomfortable it is mandatory to compare both shoulders.

The locking position should then be tested on both shoulders, feeling for and comparing the range, the intensity and the site of pain.

The normal 'feel' of these movements must be learnt if small disturbances responsible for minor yet important symptoms are not to be missed.

OTHER TEST MOVEMENTS

Flexion

In both examination and treatment, flexion must be assessed in all positions between full flexion alongside the head and the quadrant position (approximately 30 degrees lateral to the head). The position of flexion where the main limitation of range or degree of pain is felt is usually the position utilized in treatment (*Figure 6.3*).

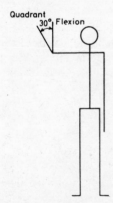

Figure 6.3. – Patient supine. Testing by overpressure on the elbow positions between flexion and the quadrant

When the glenohumeral joint has obvious limitations of active range the quadrant and locking positions are not required as part of examination.

Horizontal flexion

This is an important movement which should be assessed routinely as it can restrict certain important functional movements.

Accessory movements

The accessory movements tested as part of examination and referred to in Table 6.1 are depicted in this Chapter in *Figures 6.17–6.30.*

ASSESSMENT DURING TREATMENT

Active abduction in standing without lateral rotation is the movement commonly used for assessing progress, but when all movements of the glenohumeral joint are limited and painful it is more useful to the physiotherapist to assess active flexion. This is because if treatment effects a 5 per cent improvement, it will be more evident on assessing flexion which has a range of 180 degrees than in the smaller range of abduction.

TECHNIQUES

Flexion and quadrant***

Neither flexion nor the quadrant is used as a grade I movement in treatment for reasons already given (*see* page 19). Grades II, III and IV, however, are commonly used and the movement may be directed towards any point between full flexion and the quadrant, but it is usually directed towards the limitation or the painful position.

GRADE II***

Starting position

The physiotherapist stands beyond the patient's shoulder facing his feet. With his arm flexed, she holds his wrist and hand in her left hand. His hand does not then flap loosely during treatment. She holds his elbow in her right hand with her fingers spreading over the medial aspect of the joint reaching to the upper arm; her thumb is cupped around his forearm just distal to the elbow. She places her right knee on the couch beyond his shoulder. To prevent the movement going beyond an established range of flexion the physiotherapist must position her thigh as a stop for the patient's upper arm as it makes contact across her inner thigh. A pillow or blanket should not be used to form the stop as small variations in the range of flexion cannot properly be controlled. The further lateral elevation is directed the further from the patient's head the physiotherapist needs to stand. Balance is maintained between her standing leg (in this case the left leg) and her right lower leg (*Figure 6.4a*).

Method

The movement, which consists of raising and lowering the patient's arm through approximately 30 degrees, must be directed in a straight line. The humerus must not swing through an arc. During the treatment movement the patient's wrist traverses the same amplitude as his elbow, thus avoiding humeral rotation. If the flexion is directed towards the quadrant, the movement must be in a line from the opposite hip to the quadrant. The nearer the flexion is directed to the patient's head the more the starting position of the line is directed from the hip of the same side. With this change of treatment direction, the physiotherapist will most probably need to use the other leg to form the stop (*Figure 6.4b*).

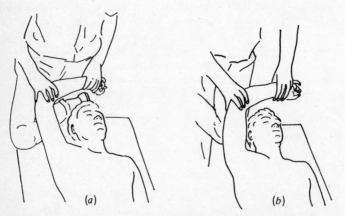

Figure 6.4 — Glenohumeral joint, grade II. (a) quadrant; (b) flexion

As pain recedes and it becomes necessary to move the arm further into the range, the physiotherapist should lower her thigh which supports his arm. At the same time she must withdraw her knee a little to prevent pressure being exerted against the upper end of the humerus as this would produce movement of the anterior head in the glenoid cavity during mobilization. In fact there are times when the anterior movement should be incorporated with the techniques. This is when glenohumeral flexion is stiff and the head of the humerus needs to be pushed longitudinally to aid gaining improvement in flexion range. Also it may be used when it is desirable to reproduce pain and the addition of the anterior movement does achieve this.

GRADE III***

Method

Patients with stiff shoulders will have the same starting position and methods for grade III as described above for grade II, with the physiotherapist's thigh providing the stop at the limit of the range. When the range is not limited, the physiotherapist stands in the same position but uses the treatment couch, not her leg, to provide the stop. When a III+ movement is used and the range of movement is good, the physiotherapist stands to the left of the patient's head and grasps his right forearm just proximal to the wrist (*Figure 6.5a*). With this grasp she oscillates his arm in the chosen position, through an amplitude of approximately 30 degrees.

If a greater range of flexion is possible the physiotherapist places her left hand under his right scapula to raise his shoulder while controlling the mobilization with her right hand (*Figure 6.5b*).

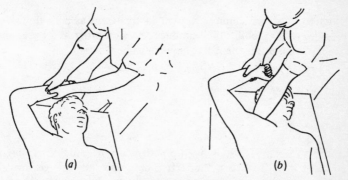

Figure 6.5. – Glenohumeral joint; quadrant, grade III

The incorporation of medial or lateral rotation can be used, as indicated by assessment and examination, to assist improvement of range (when it is stiff in the particular direction) or to reproduce pain.

GRADE IV***

Starting position

The starting position is the same as that adopted to find the quadrant position (*Figure 6.2*). The physiotherapist's nearside arm supports under the upper rib angles to raise the shoulder while she holds the patient's elbow in her left hand in a manner which controls rotation.

Method

A firm grasp of the patient's elbow is necessary when the movement is performed at the limit of range in small amplitudes. The mobilization should be performed as an oscillatory movement of 5 degrees or less (*Figure 6.2*) rather than as a sustained stretch.

As described for grade III, there are occasions when the physical findings indicate that rotation should be used in conjunction with flexion. When this is necessary, the patient's wrist does not traverse the same amplitude as the elbow but is controlled so as to rotate the humerus to the limit of the range at the moment when full flexion is reached. This can be done with medial or lateral rotation.

Abduction

Abduction is not as commonly used in treatment as is flexion. However, when other mobilizations produce only slow progress the usefulness of abduction as a treatment technique must be assessed.

GRADE II**

Starting position

The physiotherapist stands by the patient's right shoulder facing his feet. She cups the web of her left thumb and index finger over his shoulder medial to the acromion process, her fingers extending over the scapula and her thumb extending forwards over the clavicle, or uses the heel of her hand over the clavicle. With her right hand she reaches around his forearm to grasp his elbow from the medial side so that his right forearm is supported by her forearm. She stabilizes his shoulder with her left hand while she abducts his arm to the chosen angle. Her thigh, in contact with the lateral surface of his elbow, provides the stop for the movement (*Figure 6.6a*).

Alternative starting position

The physiotherapist can hold the patient's right forearm by grasping proximal to his wrist. Her index finger extends along the anterior surface of the forearm, her fingers around the medial border and her thumb around the lateral border. This position requires a tight grasp with the right hand and this may hinder relaxation. The choice of position is guided entirely by the ease with which a relaxed movement can be produced (*Figure 6.6b*).

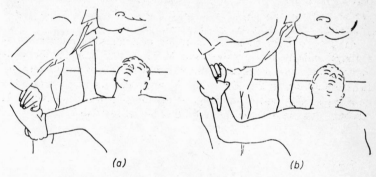

(a)   (b)

Figure 6.6. – Glenohumeral joint; abduction, grade II

Method

The patient's arm is moved from adduction until the physiotherapist's thigh stops further abduction. The movement is oscillated back and forth in the amplitude dictated by the patient's signs, usually through an arc of 20 degrees or more. Some patients find it easier to relax their arm as it is moved pendulum fashion with the forearm grasp rather than with support under the elbow. The physiotherapist's left hand should be comfortably positioned and maintain an unchanging pressure against the acromion process.

GRADE III**

The only variation from the foregoing procedure is that the physiotherapist must hold more firmly with her left hand to stabilize the
shoulder girdle when the abduction movement is taken to the limit of
the range. This pressure should be constant and not increased in such a
way as to serve as an equal and opposite counterpressure at the limit
of the abduction. It is not possible to produce grade III movement
with the forearm grasp; instead the support must be given under the
elbow.

GRADE IV**

Starting position

When the range is limited and firm stretching mobilizations are required,
the physiotherapist changes her position to stand beyond the patient's
elbow and faces his shoulder: a straight line from the patient's shoulder
to the centre of the physiotherapist's pelvis should pass slightly lateral
to the shaft of the humerus when it is abducted to the desired position.

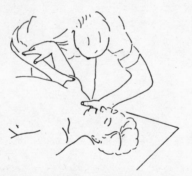

*Figure 6.7. – Glenohumeral joint; abduc-
tion, grade IV*

She then crouches over the patient's arm, places her left hand over the
acromion process and her right hand under the patient's elbow. This
technique can be used to stretch tight structures between the humerus
and the scapula on the one hand and on the other to emphasize the
downward movement of the head of the humerus in the glenoid, a
normal action which takes place during abduction of the normal

shoulder. If the physiotherapist places her left hand over the acromion process the technique will stretch the structure between the humerus and the scapula. An important change in the technique is made if she places her left hand over the head of the humerus immediately adjacent to the lateral border of the acromion process. Under these circumstances, during abduction of the shoulder, pressure from her left hand will encourage downward movement of the head of the humerus in the glenoid. Her forearms should be positioned in the coronal plane pointing in opposite directions (*Figure 6.7*).

Method

The physiotherapist's right arm produces small amplitude oscillations (two or three degrees) while her left hand maintains a constant pressure against the acromion process. The pressure of the left hand does not increase as the arm reaches the limit of abduction to give an equal and opposite counterpressure but rather allows the shoulder girdle to rise a limited amount as this allows for better relaxation.

As has been described above the counterpressure of the physiotherapist's left hand can be on the head of the humerus rather than on the acromion process. When this method is used during the abduction movement the pressure of the left hand on the head of the humerus is an equal and opposite counterpressure so as to push the head of the humerus downwards in the glenoid.

Locking position***

Starting position

When the locking position described on page 66 is the only limited movement, the starting position is the same as that described for finding the quadrant by moving the arm from abduction to flexion (*see Figure 6.1*, page 66).

Method

The mobilization consists of either an oscillatory abduction movement or a semicircular movement of the elbow. The dome of the semicircle faces superiorly and the movement is performed as if to scour out the position where the humerus should become locked. The semicircular movement of the elbow is depicted by the double-headed arrow in *Figure 6.8.*

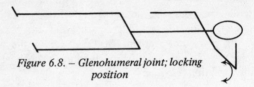

Figure 6.8. — Glenohumeral joint; locking position

Lateral rotation**

Because lateral rotation is not commonly used when pain is dominant, grades I and II— are rarely used. As very strong pressures should not be used in this direction grade IV has little application. Grade II is occasionally used and grades II+ and III— are frequently used. The rotary movement can be performed with the humerus in adduction by the patient's side, in abduction, or in any position between these two limits as dictated by the most painful position or the position exhibiting the greatest limitation.

GRADES II+ AND III—**

Grades II+ and III— differ only slightly in their end positions, with III— being slightly deeper in the range than II+. They can therefore be described together.

Starting position

The physiotherapist stands by the patient's abducted right arm, facing his feet. She cups her left hand laterally around his upper arm near the elbow with her fingers supporting posteriorly and her thumb anteriorly. She positions her left forearm as a stop to prevent his right forearm

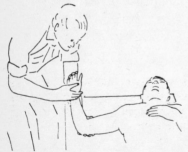

Figure 6.9. — Glenohumeral joint; lateral rotation

going further into lateral rotation than the selected range. With her right hand she grasps his slightly pronated wrist, spreading her fingers across his wrist and distal forearm anteriorly while her thumb grasps the back of his wrist (*Figure 6.9*).

Method

The oscillatory movement is produced by a to-and-fro movement of the physiotherapist's right hand through approximately 30 degrees around the arc of a circle the centre of which is his elbow. The movement is taken up to the stop provided by her left forearm. It is important that the patient's wrist should be relaxed during the movement as this will assist relaxation of his shoulder. Her cup-like grasp around his upper arm should be loose, permitting a free rotary movement while at the same time providing a stable pivot point.

If a more vigorous movement is desired, the starting position should be changed to provide greater stability.

Starting position**

The physiotherapist stands beyond the patient's right shoulder. His abducted upper arm is supported in her left hand anteriorly and inferiorly near the elbow, the point of his elbow extending beyond the edge of the couch. She uses her right thigh, appropriately placed, to form the stop at the limit of the range. She grasps his right wrist

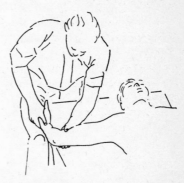

Figure 6.10. – Glenohumeral joint; lateral
rotation

with her index and middle fingers spreading proximally over his pronated wrist anteriorly while grasping through the first interosseous space with her thumb. Her remaining fingers spread around the ulnar border of his hand to reach the dorsum (*Figure 6.10*).

Method

In this position she can comfortably stabilize around the lower end of his upper arm to form the pivot for the rotation. The rotation is produced through a stable grasp of his wrist pivoting around her grasp of his upper arm. This position aids relaxation because the arm is fully supported, and the firm stop assures the patient that the movement will not be taken beyond the comfortable limit.

Medial rotation

Medial rotation is usefully employed in movements ranging from grade II with the arm either by the side or in abduction, to grade IV movements in the functional position with the arm behind the back.

GRADE II**

Starting position

The physiotherapist stands by the patient's right hip, facing his head. After abducting his arm, she supports under the distal end of his humerus with the fingers of her right hand and cups her thumb anteriorly. She grasps over the back of his hand with her left hand, her fingers spreading across the back of his wrist and her thumb grasping anteriorly. When his arm is medially rotated the anterior surface of his forearm contacts the anterior surface of her right forearm to prevent the medial rotation exceeding an established range. She can raise or lower her forearm as necessary (*Figure 6.11a*).

The physiotherapist can use her right thigh to form the stop instead of her right forearm by standing lateral to the patient's arm (*Figure 6.11b*).

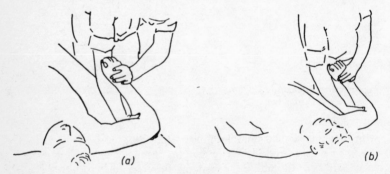

(a)   (b)

Figure 6.11. – Glenohumeral joint; medial rotation, grade II

Method

The oscillation is produced by the physiotherapist's relaxed grasp of the patient's hand. She extends his wrist slightly as the treatment movement of his forearm reaches the stop provided by her forearm or thigh. Her grasp of his upper arm in her right hand should not be tight but allow freedom of movement. If the shoulder girdle is not prevented from lifting, it provides a visual assessment of glenohumeral rotation and permits the patient a certain freedom to move if the treatment movement becomes painful.

GRADE IV**

Grade IV is not a grade of movement to be used over-enthusiastically but, as it has an occasional place in treatment, it must be described. When this grade of movement is desired the shoulder girdle must be firmly stabilized.

Starting position

The physiotherapist stands away from the right side of the patient's head facing his feet. She crouches over his right arm, abducted to the chosen range, and supports under his elbow with the fingers of her left hand from the medial side cupping her thumb anteriorly to his biceps tendon. His upper arm rests on the couch with his elbow beyond the

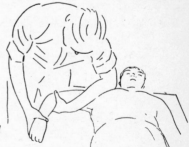

Figure 6.12. – Glenohumeral joint; medial rotation, grade IV

edge. She places her left upper arm in front of and just medial to his shoulder. With her right hand she holds his pronated wrist grasping around the ulnar border, her fingers covering the anterior surface of his wrist and adjacent palm and her thenar eminence and thumb, pointing caudally, holding over the posterior surface of his wrist (*Figure 6.12*).

Method

The small amplitude rotary oscillations of approximately 10 degrees are performed by the physiotherapist's right hand on the patient's right wrist at that point in the range which makes the patient's shoulder girdle lift. She limits the lifting of his right shoulder with her left upper arm which moves with the shoulder, providing only enough counter-pressure to prevent it lifting too far. She prevents his arm drifting into adduction. When the arm requires treatment in this position the movement is usually grade IV.

Hand behind back

The hand behind the back position, which is functionally important, is dependent upon medial rotation, extension and to some extent adduction. When the arm requires treatment in this position the movement is usually grade IV.

Starting position***

The patient lies prone, turned slightly towards his right with his right arm behind his back and the physiotherapist stands behind him.

1. If medial rotation is the component desired, she reaches across to support his elbow with her left hand by grasping posteriorly around the distal part of his upper arm. With her right hand she holds his wrist, her fingers across the posterior surface and her thumb anteriorly (*Figure 6.13a*).

2. If extension is the desired movement, she stabilizes the posterior surface of his scapula in the region of the inferior angle with her left hand and supports under his distal forearm with her right hand (*Figure 6.13b*).

3. When adduction is the movement desired, she stabilizes his scapula with her left thumb against the medial border inferiorly, and her fingers spread across the adjacent surface of the scapula. With her right hand she grasps around the patient's upper forearm (*Figure 6.13c*).

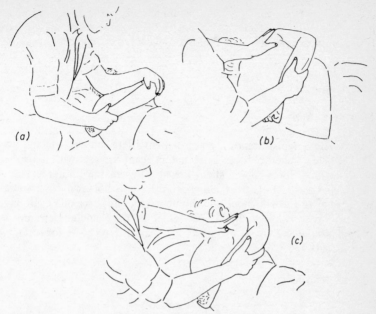

Figure 6.13. – Glenohumeral joint; hand behind the back position (a) medial rotation; (b) extension; (c) adduction

Method

In all three of the above positions the small oscillatory movement is produced by the physiotherapist's right hand. However, finer control of the adduction movement can sometimes be achieved by a lateral or postero-anterior movement of the inferior angle of the scapula. This movement is produced by her left arm acting through her left thumb against the medial border of the scapula near the inferior angle.

Although the movements of medial rotation, extension and adduction have been described separately they can be used in any combination. The choice of the combination is guided by the signs found on examination or by the progress achieved with the individual movement.

Horizontal flexion

Horizontal flexion is another movement which is not used often in treatment as a technique on its own. However, it is frequently incorporated in treatment when movements in several directions are used.

Assessment of its value as a solo technique may be necessary if treatment using other movements is not making adequate progress or if horizontal flexion is the main limitation of movement.

GRADES II AND III**

Starting position

The physiotherapist stands by the patient's left shoulder, facing his right shoulder. She holds his wrist and adjacent forearm with her right hand with his elbow and shoulder flexed 90 degrees. With her left arm she reaches across the patient and grasps the lateral border of his scapula so that her thenar eminence and thumb extend into his axilla overlying the anterior surface of the lateral border of the scapula. Her fingers extend around the lateral margin of the scapula to its posterior surface.

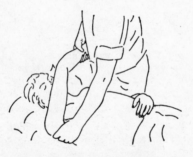

Figure 6.14. – Glenohumeral joint; horizontal flexion, grades II and III

To permit as much freedom in horizontal flexion as possible his arm is positioned midway between medial and lateral glenohumeral rotation. It is only possible to provide a stop for this movement by positioning her body to prevent his right hand continuing its movement (*Figure 6.14*).

Method

Because horizontal flexion is a difficult movement to perform smoothly in large amplitudes more care than usual is required. The physiotherapist performs it with her right arm while her left hand stabilizes his scapula.

GRADE IV**

Starting position

The physiotherapist stands by the patient's right shoulder facing across his body and places the heel of her left hand under the medial border of his right scapula at the level of the spine of the scapula. While holding his right wrist in her right hand, she flexes his elbow and shoulder and carries his arm across into horizontal flexion. She then

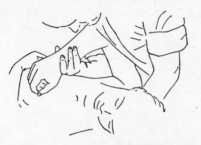

Figure 6.15. – Glenohumeral joint; horizontal flexion, grade IV

leans across the patient and places his elbow and adjacent forearm into her right anterior axillary wall. His arm, positioned midway between medial and lateral glenohumeral rotation is horizontally flexed further until scapular protraction is complete. She then corrects her left hand position against the medial border of his scapula (*Figure 6.15*).

Method

The small amplitude oscillation is produced by the physiotherapist alternately increasing and decreasing her pressure against the patient's upper arm. This pressure is transmitted to her left hand against the vertebral border of the scapula. The horizontal flexion oscillation can be produced by a two-fold action. Firstly, the pressure is directed along the line of the shaft of the humerus and this pressure will increase the range of the horizontal flexion because the heel of her left hand will hold the medial border of the scapula against the rib-cage while the lateral border will move posteriorly. Secondly, pressure is also exerted against the patient's elbow and this pressure will be directed in a line towards his opposite shoulder. When this technique is used in treatment the two directions can be used either independently or in conjunction with each other. The choice will depend upon which method produces the strongest horizontal flexion or which of the methods reproduces the patient's symptoms.

Horizontal extension

This technique is not frequently used in treatment but it can be helpful when pain arises from the acromioclavicular joint or when the patient is unable to abduct his arm without bringing it forwards from the frontal plane.

GRADE IV

Starting position

The patient lies on his back with his acromion process at the edge of the couch. The physiotherapist places her fingers under his acromion process to both feel the joint movement and protect the patient against contact with the hard and sharp edge of the couch.

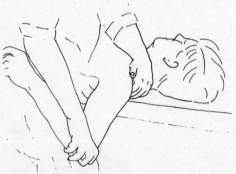

Figure 6.16. – Glenohumeral joint; hori-
zontal extension

With her other arm she holds around his elbow and stabilizes his forearm against her side or thigh.

She then pushes the patient's elbow towards the floor so as to produce horizontal extension at the glenohumeral joint (*Figure 6.16*).

Method

Having taken a patient up to the limit of his horizontal extension the physiotherapist then applies pressure in this same direction as a small amplitude oscillatory movement. The degree of abduction of the glenohumeral joint in which this horizontal extension is performed will depend upon the examination findings. If the technique is being used to relieve pain then the degree of abduction chosen would be the one which reproduced the pain. This does not mean that the treatment technique is done in a painful part of that range but it is done in that direction. If the technique is aimed at stretching the movement then the degree of abduction would be the one in which horizontal extension is most limited.

This movement can also be done as a grade II or III movement though it is most commonly performed as a grade IV movement.

Longitudinal movement caudad**

Longitudinal movement is movement of the head of the humerus from the superior extent of the glenoid cavity to its inferior extent. It can be performed with the patient's arm by his side, or with his arm in abduction, flexion or elevation.

ARM BY SIDE***

The arm by side movement can be produced either by the physiotherapist's thumbs on the head of the humerus or by a grasp around the arm. When treating a very painful joint the arm-grasp is better because the head of the humerus is too tender for direct contact. Gentle grade I movements can be very effective in the treatment of very painful glenohumeral joint conditions, and those unaccustomed to using these techniques are usually surprised to find how gently the movements must be performed and how effective the techniques then are.

Starting position (Grade I)

The physiotherapist kneels by the patient's right elbow. She flexes his elbow and holds his wrist in her right hand while gently hugging his right forearm to her with her right forearm. She places the fingers of her left hand over his upper arm with the lateral border of the proximal phalanx of her index finger against the anterior surface of the proximal end of his forearm and her thumb against the lateral surface of the elbow (*Figure 6.17a*).

Method (Grade I)

For grade I movements tiny oscillations are effected by alternating pressures against the patient's forearm through the physiotherapist's index finger. His right upper arm should be held clear of the couch to enable the movement to be free of friction. When extremely gentle techniques are being used it is essential to withdraw the index finger from the patient's forearm far enough to allow the head of the humerus

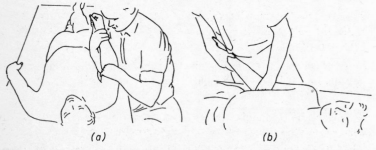

(a)   (b)

Figure 6.17. – Glenohumeral joint; longitudinal movement caudad, arm by side, grade I

to return to the superior part of the glenoid cavity. This return movement can be assisted by maintaining the patient's elbow slightly more flexed than a right angle. If the position is maintained it will be natural for the head of the humerus to move upwards in the glenoid cavity once the pressure from the left hand is released (*Figure 6.17a*). This degree of elbow flexion is not required for movements which are performed strongly and in fact a straighter arm enables the physiotherapist's right hand to assist the longitudinal movement (*Figure 6.17b*).

Starting position (Grades II, III and IV)***

Grades II, III and IV are performed with very similar starting positions with the variations in amplitude and depth of range being controlled by the physiotherapist.

When direct pressure is used against the head of the humerus the physiotherapist stands beyond the patient's head at the right side and places the pads of her thumbs against the head of the humerus immediately adjacent to the anterior and lateral borders of the acromion

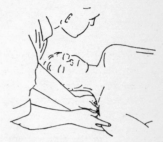

Figure 6.18. – Glenohumeral joint; longitudinal movement caudad, arm by side, grades II, III and IV

process. The fingers of her left hand are spread over the scapular area while the fingers of her right hand spread laterally over the deltoid (*Figure 6.18*).

Method (Grades II, III and IV)

To make the technique more comfortable for the patient, and to enable the physiotherapist to feel the movement of the head of the humerus in relation to the acromion process, the oscillatory movement is produced by the physiotherapist's arms, not by the intrinsic muscles of the thumbs.

IN ABDUCTION***

The abduction technique is used only when the joint condition requires movement ranging from II+ to IV+.

Starting position

The physiotherapist stands by the patient's right shoulder facing across his body. She abducts his right arm with her right hand while supporting his elbow at a right angle. She supports the distal end of his upper arm medially and posteriorly with the fingers of her right hand while her thumb extends anteriorly around his elbow. Her wrist rests against the anteromedial surface of his forearm and his forearm is supported by her right forearm. The heel of her left hand is placed against the head of his humerus immediately adjacent to the acromion

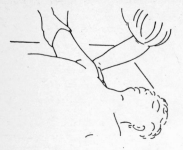

Figure 6.19. – Glenohumeral joint; longitudinal movement in abduction

process and her fingers spread over his shoulder towards his neck. For stronger techniques it is necessary to crouch over the patient's arm so that her left forearm, directed caudally, lies in the coronal plane (*Figure 6.19*).

Method

The movement is produced entirely by the pressure of the physiotherapist's left hand against the head of the humerus.

The movement can be performed in two different ways. The first is that as she exerts pressure against the head of the humerus, moving it towards the patient's feet, she can carry his elbow so that the elbow moves as far longitudinally as does the shoulder girdle. Secondly, she can hold his elbow stationary while applying longitudinal movement to the head of the humerus. This latter technique results in longitudinal movement of the head of the humerus in the glenoid cavity combined with a small degree of abduction of the glenohumeral joint brought about by keeping the elbow stationary.

The movement of the head of the humerus can be felt in relation to the stationary acromion process.

IN ABDUCTION PRONE**

The abduction prone technique for this movement has the advantage of stabilizing the patient's arm more firmly and leaving the physiotherapist's two hands free both to control and feel the amount of accessory movement available in the joint.

Starting position

The patient lies prone with his arm abducted and laterally rotated. If the joint range is limited the patient will need to lie more on his left side so that his shoulder will not be extended. The physiotherapist stands by the right side of his head facing his feet. She places her two

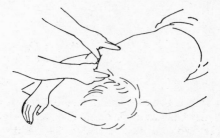

Figure 6.20. – Glenohumeral joint; longitudinal movement in abduction prone

thumbs against the head of the humerus immediately adjacent to the acromion process with her fingers spread over the anterior deltoid and lateral scapular area. She then directs her arms caudally in line with the longitudinal movement of the head of the humerus (*Figure 6.20*).

Method

The oscillatory movement is produced from the physiotherapist's body and arms acting through her thumbs. It must not be produced by the thumb flexors. If gentle movements are required, the point of contact should be through the tips of the thumbs. As stronger movements are desired more of the pad should be brought into contact with the head of the humerus.

IN 90 DEGREES FLEXION***

The movement in flexion is usually only required as one of a number of techniques used to mobilize generally a moderately painful or stiff joint.

Starting position

The physiotherapist stands by the patient's right shoulder facing across his body and supports his right arm, flexed to 90 degrees at the shoulder and elbow, with her right arm. She supports his wrist in her right hand, his forearm on her forearm, and his upper arm against her side. The

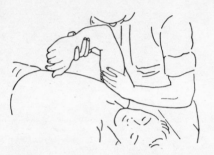

Figure 6.21. – Glenohumeral joint; longitudinal movement in 90 degrees flexion

glenohumeral joint is positioned midway between medial and lateral rotation. Her left hand is placed against the head of the humerus just distal to the acromion process with her fingers directed distally. Her thumb extends laterally round his upper arm (*Figure 6.21*).

Method

The oscillatory longitudinal movement is produced by pressure against the head of the humerus with the heel of the left hand. The physiotherapist's right hand supports the patient's arm and carries it with the movement so that the angle of flexion at the shoulder is not altered. Alternatively if she holds the elbow stationary a small degree of flexion at the glenohumeral joint will accompany the longitudinal movement.

IN FULL FLEXION***

The movement in flexion is of particular use as a grade IV mobilization. It has no place in the treatment of shoulders which are limited in range by pain as the pain would increase unnecessarily.

Starting position

The physiotherapist stands by the patient's right side beyond his head. She crouches over his shoulder and holds his flexed right arm against her left side. She then places her hands together, behind his deltoid, with the posterior surface of her left index finger against the anterior

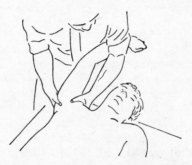

*Figure 6.22. – Glenohumeral joint; longi-
tudinal movement in full flexion*

surface of her right index finger and the lateral surfaces against the head of the humerus immediately adjacent to the acromion process. Her thumbs extend around the sides of his arm to point towards each other across the axilla. She then has a firm grasp of the upper end of the humerus near the surgical neck (*Figure 6.22*).

Method

Before performing the oscillation the physiotherapist applies pressure through the lateral border of her index fingers to take up the slack by raising the shoulder girdle and moving it caudally. Once this slack has been taken up the oscillation can be performed by alternately increasing and decreasing further pressure to direct the head of the humerus distally in the glenoid cavity.

Postero-anterior movement***

The postero-anterior movement is one of the most valuable movements in the treatment of extremely painful shoulders. It is not a technique which is hindered by local tenderness as is longitudinal movement. Grade I movements are better produced by direct thumb pressures against the head of the humerus than by using the upper arm as a lever because of the difference in the accuracy of control possible with each method.

Starting position

The patient lies with his elbow flexed and his forearm resting against his trunk. If he finds it uncomfortable with his shoulder in this degree of glenohumeral extension a pillow or blanket should be placed under his elbow. When this change is made a pillow must also be placed on his abdomen to support his forearm so that medial rotation of the glenohumeral joint is avoided. The physiotherapist kneels laterally and superiorly to the patient's shoulder and positions her two thumbs, back to back, with their tips in contact with the posterior surface of the head of the humerus adjacent to the acromion process. The fingers of her left hand are spread over the clavicular area and those of her right hand spread over the deltoid (*Figure 6.23*).

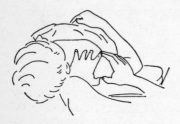

Figure 6.23. – *Glenohumeral joint; postero-anterior movement*

Method

It is of prime importance that the oscillatory movement should be produced by the physiotherapist's arms. If the movement is produced by the thumb flexors the movement becomes uncomfortable for the patient and the physiotherapist loses all feel of movement.

When grades I and II movements are used it is imperative that there should be no pressure against the head of the humerus at the beginning of the movement and that, with each oscillation, the head of the humerus is returned to this relaxed position. As the pressure will be very light the points of the thumbs should be used.

When stronger movements are required (grades III and IV) it is advisable to change the point of contact from the tips of the thumbs to a larger area of the pads. This anteriorly directed movement of the head of the humerus can be further emphasized by an anteroposterior pressure against the clavicle with the little and ring fingers of the left hand.

Alternative starting position**

When pain is minimal and both accessory and physiological movements are used to mobilize the joint, it may be more suitable to use the patient's arm as a lever. This change involves a completely different technique.

The physiotherapist stands by the patient's right forearm facing his head. She holds his forearm against her right side and supports

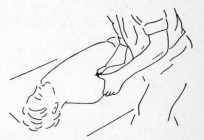

Figure 6.24. – Glenohumeral joint; postero-anterior movement

under the posterior surface of the head of the humerus with a similar hand grip to that described for 'longitudinal movement in full flexion' (*see* page 91). The posterior surface of the right hand is placed in the palmar surface of the left hand so that the index fingers overlap and the lateral borders of the index fingers contact the back of the head of the humerus. Her thumbs hold around the humerus to form an encompassing grasp. She may need to crouch to position his upper arm in the coronal plane (*Figure 6.24*).

Method

The slack of scapular movement is taken up by lifting the head of the humerus so that any further oscillatory movement will be associated with the postero-anterior glenohumeral movement. Grade III+ movements are performed like a flick, allowing the shoulder girdle to drop an inch or two before countering it with a postero-anterior pressure returning it through the same few inches. A grade IV+ mobilization is a sustained oscillatory mobilization of small amplitude at the limit of the range.

IN ABDUCTION***

Treatment in the abduction position is used as grades III or IV when pain is not severe and restoration of range is the primary factor.

Starting position

The physiotherapist stands away from the patient's right shoulder facing across his body. His straight arm is abducted and stabilized by holding his forearm against her right side. It may be necessary for her to crouch to position his arm in the coronal plane. The grasp is the same as that described for *Figure 6.24* (*Figure 6.25*).

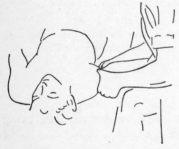

Figure 6.25. – Glenohumeral joint; postero-anterior movement in ab-duction

Method

The movements for grade III and grade IV are performed in an identical manner to that described for producing postero-anterior movements using the patient's arms as a lever (*see* page 93). Care must be exercised when taking up the slack of scapulothoracic movement.

IN ABDUCTION PRONE**

This alternative position provides a greater feel for grade IV movements and leaves the physiotherapist free to use both hands to control the accessory movement.

Starting position

The patient lies prone with his arm abducted and laterally rotated. If the joint range is limited the patient will need to turn slightly towards his right so that his shoulder will not be extended. The physiotherapist stands by his right shoulder facing across his body and places the pads

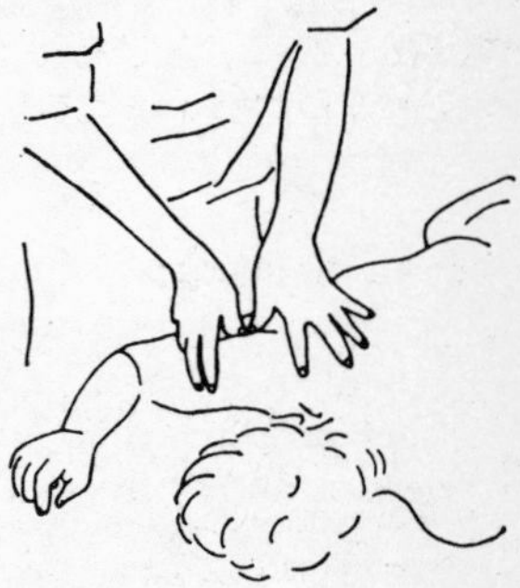

Figure 6.26. – Glenohumeral joint; postero-anterior movement in abduction prone

of both thumbs against the posterior surface of the head of the humerus immediately adjacent to the acromion process. She then directs her arms in a postero-anterior direction with her shoulders positioned immediately above the direction of the movement (*Figure 6.26*).

Method

The mobilization is produced by the physiotherapist's arms acting through a spring-like action of the thumbs. The flexors of the thumbs must not produce the movement because the technique then becomes uncomfortable and the thumbs will not be able to appreciate small glenohumeral movements.

IN FULL FLEXION***

This movement is of particular use as a grade IV mobilization; it has no place in the treatment of very painful shoulder conditions. The starting position is identical with that described for 'longitudinal movement in full flexion' (*see* page 90). The difference in the method lies in the direction of the oscillation; the head of the humerus is directed anteriorly in the glenoid cavity, not longitudinally.

Anteroposterior movement**

ARM BY SIDE**

This anteroposterior movement is not as useful as 'longitudinal movement' or 'postero-anterior movement' in the treatment of very painful shoulders. Its main application in treatment lies more in grades III and IV when the joint is stiff and moderately painful.

Starting position

The physiotherapist stands by the patient's right upper arm facing across his body. With the fingers of her right hand she supports the lower end of his humerus posteriorly from the medial side and then rests his forearm on her forearm. She raises his upper arm approximately 10 degrees anteriorly to the coronal plane of the trunk and rests his

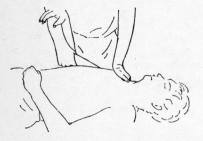

Figure 6.27. – Glenohumeral joint; anteroposterior movement arm by side

forearm against her forearm. This position allows a better anteroposterior movement of the head of the humerus in the glenoid. She places the heel of her left hand anteriorly over the head of the humerus with her fingers extending superiorly and posteriorly over the acromion process (*Figure 6.27*).

Method

The anteroposterior oscillation is produced by pressure of the heel of her left hand against the head of the humerus. Her fingers, cupped loosely around the acromion process, do not apply any pressure but assist in feeling the movement. Different degrees of pressure are required for different grades of movement and greater recoil is permitted for the larger amplitudes.

IN ABDUCTION***

This movement is only applicable when treatment requires grades III and IV movements.

Starting position

The physiotherapist stands by the patient's right shoulder, facing his feet. She supports the distal end of his humerus posteriorly from the

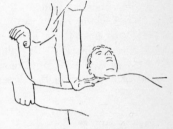

Figure 6.28. – Glenohumeral joint; anteroposterior movement in abduction

medial side with her right hand, abducts his arm then rests his flexed forearm on her forearm. She places the heel of her left hand anteriorly against the head of his humerus with her fingers extending medially across the adjacent clavicular area (*Figure 6.28*).

Method

The oscillatory movement is produced by pressure against the head of the humerus with her left hand.

It may be found that the anteroposterior movement is more effective in different degrees of glenohumeral extension or horizontal flexion. Anteroposterior movement in the different positions in this horizontal plane should be assessed to find the stiffest or most painful part of the movement before using the technique as a mobilization. This searching for the relevant sign is used with all techniques and is fundamental to effective treatment.

IN HORIZONTAL FLEXION**

The horizontal flexion position is only used when general mobilization is being employed for a stiff joint. Only grades III and IV therefore are likely to be used. The starting position is similar to that described for horizontal flexion (*see* page 83). The difference is that the humerus is vertical and the hand under the scapula is placed laterally. The antero-posterior movement is produced by pressure directed down the shaft of the humerus.

Lateral movement

As with all passive accessory movement (except longitudinal movement and postero-anterior movement with the arm by the side), this technique has its main value in the restoration of range rather than in the treatment of the very painful joint which the patient is unable to move because of pain. It is therefore one of many accessory movements used in combination with others in treatment. The movement is performed in two basic positions; one with the arm by the side and the other with the arm in 90 degrees of flexion.

ARM BY SIDE***

Starting position

The physiotherapist stands by the patient's right side distal to his flexed elbow facing his head. She places her right hand as high as possible to his axilla with her palm in contact with the medial surface of his humerus. Her fingers spread posteriorly around his arm while her thumb crosses the anterior deltoid. Her left hand supports his

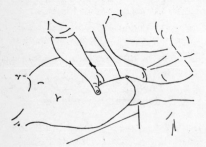

Figure 6.29. – Glenohumeral joint; lateral movement arm by side

elbow, the palm of her hand against the lateral surface of the joint and her fingers supporting posteriorly. She then crouches over his arm so that her forearms can be directed opposite each other in as near the coronal plane as possible (*Figure 6.29*).

Method

The mobilization is effected by pressure through her right hand against the upper end of the humerus. If a grade III movement is desired, her pressure must be almost completely released at the end of each oscillation. During grade IV movements, however, some pressure is maintained throughout the technique while an increase and decrease of this pressure produces the oscillation.

IN FLEXION**

Starting position

The physiotherapist stands distal to the patient's right shoulder, facing his head. She grasps the distal end of his upper arm laterally with the fingers of her left hand across the biceps and her thumb across the triceps. With this grasp she flexes his glenohumeral joint 90 degrees,

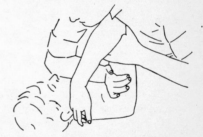

Figure 6.30. – Glenohumeral joint; lateral movement in flexion

allowing his elbow to relax comfortably in flexion. She places her right hand against the medial surface of the upper end of his humerus, high in the axilla with her fingers and thumb spreading anteriorly. By crouching over his arm she can point her forearm in opposite directions in the horizontal and coronal planes (*Figure 6.30*).

Method

Movements are produced by her right arm while her left hand either stabilizes the position of his humerus in relation to the scapula by following the movement of the head of the humerus, or it does the opposite by moving the elbow medially. The choice depends on the pain or stiffness found on examination of the movement and the intention to relieve pain or stretch stiffness.

SCAPULOTHORACIC MOVEMENT

It is uncommon for scapulothoracic movements to be painful or restricted unless the history includes trauma. The techniques therefore are not commonly used in treatment, but are techniques, which the

Table 6.2
Scapulothoracic Movement: Objective Examination

Observation

Active movements
Active quick tests (glenohumeral, cervical and thoracic)
Routinely
1. Glenohumeral (G/H) F, Ab, behind back, HF
2. Scapular elevation, depression, protraction and retraction
Note range, pain and scapular rhythm
As applicable
Speed of test movements
Specific movements which aggravate
The injuring movement
Movements under load
Muscle power

Static tests
Rotator cuff
Other muscles in 'plan'

Other joints in 'plan'

Passive movements
Physiological movements
Routinely
1. G/H movements
2. Side lying, scapular elevation, depression, protraction and rotation
Note range, pain, resistance, spasm and behaviour

Accessory movements
Routinely
Lifting scapula off thorax
Note range, pain, resistance, spasm and behaviour

Palpation

Check case records etc.

HIGHLIGHT MAIN FINDINGS WITH ASTERISKS

After treatment

physiotherapist must be able to handle, even if they are only used for examination purposes (Table 6.2). When treatment is necessary the type of movement involved is usually a grade III or IV in the direction of the painful limitation. The movements are protraction, retraction, elevation, depression and rotation.

Protraction**

Starting position

The patient lies on his left side near the forward edge of the couch, his head resting on pillows and his hips and knees comfortably flexed. The physiotherapist stands by his hips, facing his head, and leans across his pelvis to cradle his right ilium in her left axilla. This position aids stability during the large amplitude scapulothoracic movement. She grasps the medial border of his scapula with the fingers of her left hand.

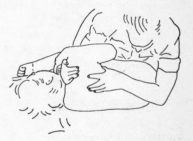

Figure 6.31. – Scapulothoracic movement; protraction

With her right hand she grasps over the spine of the scapula and cups the heel of her hand anteriorly over the clavicular area. The patient's right arm, flexed at the elbow, must be firmly supported by her right forearm to prevent any glenohumeral movement during the scapulothoracic movement (*Figure 6.31*).

Method

The protraction movement, which follows the curve of the rib cage, is produced by the fingers of both hands against the medial border and spine of the scapula. As the scapula moves around the chest wall the physiotherapist lowers the level of her support under his right arm to avoid glenohumeral movement.

Retraction**

Starting position

This position is identical with that used for protraction with one exception: the physiotherapist places her left thumb and thenar eminence very firmly along the lateral border of the scapula (*Figure 6.32*).

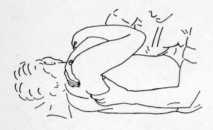

Figure 6.32. – Scapulothoracic movement; retraction

Method

Retraction is produced by pressure from the physiotherapist's grasp of the upper scapula and her left thumb against the lateral border of the scapula. Care must be exercised during the movement to see that the patient's arm is carried outwards with the scapula to avoid glenohumeral movement.

Elevation and depression**

Starting position

The starting position for these two movements is identical with that already described above except that the physiotherapist's left hand is placed over the lower half of the patient's scapula with her fingers

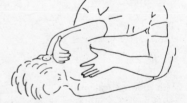

Figure 6.33 – Scapulothoracic movement; elevation and depression

pointing towards his head. The lower third of his scapula is cupped in her left hand so that her thenar eminence and thumb grasp the lateral border and her middle finger grasps the medial border (*Figure 6.33*).

Method

During the elevation the upward movement is produced by the physiotherapist's left hand and during depression it is her right hand, cupped
over the shoulder girdle, which produces it. The glenohumeral joint is
easily stabilized during both elevation and depression.

Rotation**

Starting position

The patient lies on his left side near the forward edge of the couch
with pillows to support his head. The physiotherapist stands in front
of his pelvis and with her right hand she holds over his acromial area
from in front. She flexes his right arm and rests it on her right arm.
His arm must be firmly supported to avoid glenohumeral movement
taking place during the scapulothoracic movement. With her left hand
she grasps the medial and lateral borders of the scapula with her fingers
and thumb respectively (*Figure 6.34a*).

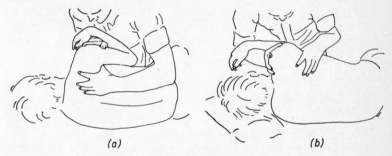

(a) (b)

Figure 6.34. – Scapulothoracic movement; rotation

Method

Scapular rotation is produced by a combined action of the physiotherapist's two hands. With her left hand she moves the inferior angle
of the scapula around the thorax while her right hand pivots the scapula
from on top. During this pivoting action her right hand stabilizes the
shoulder girdle to prevent protraction. The patient's right arm must be
stably supported on her left arm and must be flexed in unison with the
scapular movement to prevent any glenohumeral movement, and this is
in part achieved by pivoting her hips from left to right. The position at
the limit of the scapular rotation is shown in *Figure 6.34b*.

ACROMIOCLAVICULAR JOINT

The movements described for scapulothoracic movement all involve movement of the acromioclavicular joint and therefore both must be examined (Table 6.3). It is surprising, however, how infrequently

Table 6.3
Acromioclavicular Joint: Objective Examination

[When examining the acromioclavicular (A/C) joint the glenohumeral (G/H) joint must also be examined]

Observation

Active movements
  Active quick tests G/H, scap/thoracic (+cervical)
  Routinely
    1. G/H F, Ab, Behind back, HF and HE
    2. Scapular elevation, depression, protraction, retraction and rotation
  Note range, pain, repeated (note scapular rhythm)
  As applicable
    Speed of test movements
    Specific movements which aggravate
    The injuring movement
    Movements under load

Static tests
  Rotator cuff
  Other muscles in 'plan'

Other joints in 'plan'

Passive movements
Physiological movements
  Routinely
    1. G/H F, ↺ , ↻ HF and HE or quadrant and locking position
    2. Scapular elevation, depression, protraction, retraction and rotation
  Note range, pain, resistance, spasm and behaviour
Accessory movements
  Routinely
    1. By thumb pressures ↕ , ↕ ,↔ cephalad, caudad
      (*a*) over acromion
      (*b*) over clavicle
      (*c*) on the joint line
    2. Squeeze clavicle and scapula
    3. As for glenohumeral joint

Palpation

Check case records etc.

HIGHLIGHT MAIN FINDINGS WITH ASTERISKS

After treatment

these scapulothoracic movements reproduce acromioclavicular joint pain. However, pain is readily reproduced during horizontal flexion, horizontal extension, and flexion. Flexion of the glenohumeral joint is a technique frequently used in the treatment of the acromioclavicular joint. Other techniques which are more localized to the acromioclavicular joint remain to be described. One such technique involves moving the spine of the scapula and the clavicle towards each other. The remainder involve direct pressure, posteriorly, anteriorly and superiorly, against the acromial end of the clavicle.

Anteroposterior movement**

Starting position

The physiotherapist stands by the patient's right shoulder and places the heel of her left hand under the spine of his scapula near its vertebral

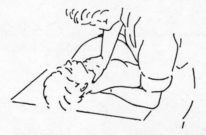

Figure 6.35. – Acromioclavicular joint; anteroposterior movement (squeeze)

end pointing her fingers towards the vertebral column. She then places the heel of her right hand over the anterior border of the clavicle near the junction of its middle and lateral thirds pointing her fingers medially (*Figure 6.35*).

Method

Movement is produced by an anteroposterior pressure against the clavicle through the heel of the physiotherapist's right hand countered by the postero-anterior pressure over the medial end of the spine of the scapula.

Alternative starting position**

This method allows for more localized technique.

   The physiotherapist stands by the patient's right shoulder, facing his head, and places her thumbs, tip to tip, against the anterior border of the clavicle immediately adjacent to the acromioclavicular joint. Her fingers are spread to provide stability. She then positions her shoulders above her hands to line up with the anteroposterior movement of the joint (*Figure 6.36*).

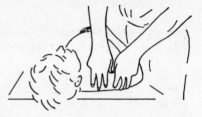

Figure 6.36. − Acromioclavicular joint; anteroposterior movement. Alternative starting position

Method

The direction of her pressure must be carefully chosen and the mobilization must be produced by her arms acting through her thumbs, not by the flexor muscles of the thumbs.

Postero-anterior movement***

Starting position

The patient rests his elbows and clasps his hands across his abdomen. The physiotherapist kneels by the right side of his head, facing his feet, and places her thumbs, tip to tip, against the posterior border of the lateral end of the clavicle. She should place as much of the pads of her thumbs as possible adjacent to the joint (*Figure 6.37*).

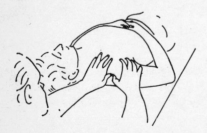

Figure 6.37. − Acromioclavicular joint; postero-anterior movement

Method

The postero-anterior movement is produced by the physiotherapist's arms acting through her thumbs. She should position her metacarpophalangeal joints close together so that the line from her shoulders to her thumbs passes through them. The movement must not be produced by the thumb flexors.

Longitudinal movement***

Longitudinal movement is so named because the movement is in line with longitudinal movement of the glenohumeral joint.

Starting position

The physiotherapist stands by the right side of the patient's head, facing his feet. She places the tips of both thumbs on the superior surface of the clavicle adjacent to the acromioclavicular joint and spreads her fingers around her thumbs to provide stability. She should

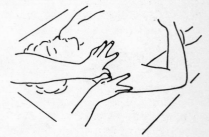

Figure 6.38. – Acromioclavicular joint; longitudinal movement caudad

position the metacarpophalangeal joints of her thumbs as close as possible to each other. Her forearms must be directed in line with the longitudinal movement of the acromioclavicular joint (*Figure 6.38*).

Method

The oscillatory mobilization is produced by her arms acting through stable thumbs. She should be able to feel movement through the base of the pad of her right thumb, which just overlies the joint, and can compare the movement of the clavicle with the stationary acromion process.

STERNOCLAVICULAR JOINT

All the movements described above for the acromioclavicular joint, together with glenohumeral flexion and all scapulothoracic movements, involve movement of the sternoclavicular joint and must be examined (Table 6.4). Localized mobilization can also be effected at this joint by thumb pressure against the sternal end of the clavicle. The technique will be described for one direction of movement only but mention will be made of the remaining movements.

Table 6.4
Sternoclavicular Joint: Objective Examination

[When examining the sternoclavicular (S/C) joint the A/C joint (including relevant G/H movements) must also be examined]

Observation

Active movements
    Active quick tests G/H and A/C (+Cervical)
    Routinely
        1. G/H F, HF and HE
        2. Scapular elevation, depression, protraction, retraction and rotation
        Note range, pain and repeated

Static tests

Other joints in 'plan'

Passive movements
Physiological movements
    Routinely
        1. Supine: G/H HF, HE, and F
        2. Side lying: Scapular elevation, depression, protraction, retraction and rotation
        Note range, pain, resistance, spasm and behaviour
Accessory movements
    Routinely
        By thumb pressures
            $\uparrow$, $\downarrow$, ◄──► caudad and cephalad, distraction
        Note range, pain, resistance, spasm and behaviour
    As applicable
        Add compression to above

Palpation

Check case records etc.

HIGHLIGHT MAIN FINDINGS WITH ASTERISKS

After treatment

Anteroposterior movement***

Starting position

The physiotherapist stands beyond the left side of the patient's head, facing his feet. She places the tips of her thumbs, pointing towards each other, directly over the sternal end of the clavicle immediately adjacent to the joint. Her fingers fan around the thumbs to provide stability.

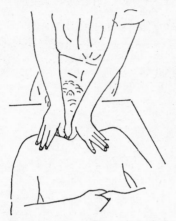

Figure 6.39. – Sternoclavicular joint; anteroposterior movement

The metacarpophalangeal joints of the thumbs are brought together so that the line of the pressure from the shoulders to the thumb tips will pass through them. It is necessary for her to position her shoulders in line with the anteroposterior movement of the joint (*Figure 6.39*).

Method

The mobilization is produced by the physiotherapist's arms and body, and must not under any circumstances be produced by the flexor muscles of the thumbs. This fact has been mentioned before but it is even more important in the sternoclavicular joint. If fine control of the movement is to be possible, and if the degree of movement is to be clearly felt, the thumbs must only transmit the pressure and not produce it. It is because this joint has such a small range of movement that the finesse with which the technique is performed is so important.

Variations .

Mobilization in a caudad direction, towards the patient's feet, can be effected by altering the point of contact to the superior surface of the medial end of the clavicle and by directing the physiotherapist's arms caudally. There is very little movement in this direction but occasionally it is more painful than other movements. It may then be the direction chosen for the treatment though it may not necessarily be performed in the painful part of the range.

When movement in the opposite direction is required, that is in a cephalad direction, the physiotherapist stands by his right elbow, facing his head. She places her thumbs against the inferior surface of the clavicle adjacent to the sternoclavicular joint. With her forearms lowered to the required angle the oscillatory movement is produced by shoulder and arm movement transmitted through her thumbs (*Figure 6.40*).

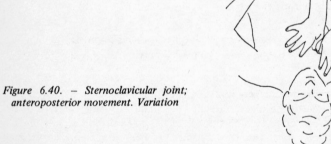

Figure 6.40. – Sternoclavicular joint; anteroposterior movement. Variation

Postero-anterior movement*

A postero-anterior movement can be produced by hooking the fingers and thumb around the medial end of the clavicle to reach its posterior surface. The movement is then produced by pulling the clavicle forwards.

In the examination of the various joints which make up shoulder girdle movements there is considerable overlap of test movements. Tables have been given for each joint. Table 6.5 aims to bring these together. It remains essential to know which joints are being tested with each individual test movement.

Table 6.5
Composite Shoulder: Objective Examination

Observation

Active quick tests
    F (spontaneous then sagittal)
    Ab (spontaneous then frontal)
    HF
    Behind back (wrist mid line)

Static tests
    Cuff

Other joints in 'plan'

Passive movements
As indicated by site of pain and stiffness
Supine
    1. G/H joint
       Q and locking position
          or
       F, Ab, ↻ ↺ , HF, HE

       Arm by side, ↕ , ↕ , ↔ caudad, ← (gapping G/H joint)
       Arm abducted, ↔ , ↕ caudad, ↕ , ↕
       Arm in F/Q ↕ , ↔ caudad
    2. A/C joint: Squeeze ↕ , ↕ , ↔ caudad and cephalad
    3. S/C joint: As applicable ↔ ceph, caud, ↕ , ↕ , distraction
Prone
    Hand behind back, E, Ad, ↻
    (forehead resting in palms,   G/H; ↕ , ↔ caudad)
Side lying
    Scap/thoracic; as applicable EL, DE, PR, RE, Rot^n

Palpation

Check case records etc.

HIGHLIGHT MAIN FINDINGS WITH ASTERISKS

After treatment

Compression and distraction

The techniques described for the sternoclavicular joint have been shown with the joint in a relaxed position. From the point of view of both examination and treatment, the same movements can be performed while the joint surfaces are compressed. The compression is produced by the physiotherapist grasping around the patient's head of humerus and acromion process and directing a pressure in line with the shaft of the clavicle. This compression can be applied at two extremes of sterno-clavicular movement, or at any position between these extremes. The first extreme is to elevate the patient's shoulder girdle, thus directing the compressive force more towards the patient's opposite hip. The other extreme is to depress the patient's shoulder girdle as much as possible, altering the angle between the clavicle and sternum so that the compressive force has a slight cephalad direction.

It is equally important to realize that the movements can also be performed when the joint surfaces are distracted. The latter technique merely requires the physiotherapist to place one hand on the medial surface of the humerus near its head and then to pull the humerus (and thus the whole shoulder girdle) laterally. As described above for compression, different angles of distraction can be used by elevating or depressing the shoulder girdle.

Both distraction and compression can be used as test movements and mobilizing techniques without being performed in conjunction with the techniques described in the text. Compression is usually of more value than distraction.

TREATMENT

The majority of patients with shoulder disorders who are referred for physiotherapy have stiffness and pain with arm movement. When examining these patients it is important to test the muscles which make up the rotator cuff as well as the ranges of movement of the individual joints to determine the muscular and capsular components of the pain. For example, it is surprising how frequently a patient with a diagnosis of 'supraspinatus tenderness' is found to have a gleno-humeral joint component also. Even when the diagnosis of supraspinatus tendonitis can be made, testing the quadrant and locking positions usually reproduces the patient's symptoms.

SUPRASPINATUS TENDONITIS

There are two methods for treating this condition by passive movement. Assuming that the quadrant and locking positions reproduce the pain, the first choice would be postero-anterior pressures against the head of the humerus with the patient's elbows by his side and his hands clasped loosely across his abdomen (*see Figure 6.23*, page 92). Initially the movements would be performed so as to avoid any pain or discomfort. Usually, the patient notices the pain recede within two or three treatments and then the amplitude of the treatment movement can be increased, reaching a painless grade III movement. Unless there has been a tear involving the tendon of the supraspinatus, the power of abduction recovers as dramatically as the pain recedes. The postero-anterior movements should be gentle to begin with and if the assessment is made carefully enough, the value of this approach will be quickly evident. It could be expected that progress would enable full amplitude, gentle, slow, oscillatory movements to be performed rocking the head of the humerus from a fully posterior position to a fully anterior position.

If the above techniques do not produce improvement quickly the quadrant movement techniques should be used, performed very gently as grade IV— movements, done either painlessly or with the least possible discomfort (*see Figure 6.2*, page 67). Assessment of their value is possible after two applications of this technique at the one treatment session. The arc of pain on abduction should improve markedly if the technique achieves the improvement expected and the power of abduction should improve also. This method of treating supraspinatus tendonitis is quicker in its effect and less painful than transverse friction massage.

FROZEN SHOULDER
FIRST STAGE

In the early stage of this clearly defined syndrome, pain is the dominant factor and the patient has little excursion of shoulder movement in any direction. Effective treatment by postero-anterior pressures can be given (*see Figure 6.23*, page 92) with the patient's arm supported on pillows in a neutral position. Great care should be taken to ensure the technique is completely painless and used only for a very short time (30 seconds). At the first treatment the physiotherapist should not assess the joint movements; assessment should be made over a 24-hour period in these early stages. The patient should experience lessening of symptoms after two treatments, enabling the physiotherapist to increase the amplitude of her technique and before long to carry the amplitude into a small degree of pain. Standing the patient and asking him to raise his arms forwards in flexion in the sagittal plane should be used for assessment; quite dramatic improvement in range of movement can be anticipated. The stages of treatment progression for pain are detailed in Chapter 5, pages 47 to 50.

SECOND STAGE

In a later stage of the untreated frozen shoulder the patient usually has painful limitation of range, and when the stiff movement is stretched, considerable pain is provoked. When both pain and stiffness are present, the initial method is to treat pain as described previously, going through the stages of accessory and physiological movements. If this approach does not produce improvement, and it should be possible to determine this within two or three treatments, then the resistance itself must be treated. The initial movement should be towards the quadrant. The physiotherapist must clearly understand how firmly she is stretching the supportive structures of the glenohumeral joint and how much pain she is provoking; on releasing the stretch she must determine how quickly the patient's pain subsides. Provided the symptoms subside immediately the stretch is released, more treatment and stronger treatment can be given.

Treatment of resistance with grade IV and grade IV+ techniques should be interspersed with movement in exactly the same direction but performed as a large amplitude grade III— technique. This will lessen treatment soreness considerably. Alternatively, large amplitude postero-anterior movement (*Figure 6.23,* page 92) is sometimes more successful in relieving treatment soreness.

It is quite common to reach a stage when the stretching movements (*Figure 6.2,* as a grade IV movement, page 67), combined with the accessory movements as described on page 91, *Figure 6.22* and on page 95, no longer produce improvement. Even with the inclusion of active exercises undertaken diligently by the patient the range may not improve. The decision has then to be made whether or not stronger pressure should be applied, assessing the strength of the resistance and the degree of pain. The patient's temperament should be taken into account and knowledge of the history of the disorder is of value in making the decision. The longer the condition has been in evidence and the less irritable it is, the safer it will be to stretch strongly. After three treatments an attempt to break adhesions may be attempted. Such manipulative procedure is in line with the MUA (manipulation under anaesthesia) procedure used by orthopaedic surgeons. Manipulation carried out on the conscious patient is preferred by some orthopaedic surgeons because under these conditions the patient's reactions can more successfully guide the manipulator.

Rarely is manipulation done at a first consultation. The technique is begun gently and repeated several times, gradually increasing in strength, the patient's reaction being watched closely meanwhile. Considerable information can be gained by watching the patient's hands and eyes.

The amount of pain the patient experiences while the structures are being stretched is estimated, thereby calculating how much pain the patient will tolerate if manipulation is attempted. Note is also taken of the strength required to increase the range. Upon release of the stretch, the time the pain or discomfort takes to subside should be ascertained. If the pain lasts for some considerable time then the physiotherapist knows she is limited in how far she can stretch and how many stretches she can apply at one session. In this way she gradually feels her way from treatment to treatment before attempting to manipulate the joint.

The movement used for manipulation is to stretch towards the quadrant position or towards full flexion alongside the patient's head, depending upon which is the stiffer and more painful. It is likely that whichever is the more painful will also be the stiffer one and therefore the more successful direction in which to manipulate. The technique used is shown in *Figure 6.2* (page 67), except that the physiotherapist will need to stabilize the patient's chest with her shoulder and trunk so that she will be in the best position to control the technique. Some manipulators consider that the manipulation should be painless and that the accessory movement should be the movement used, not the physiological movement. However the author believes that the physiological movement is usually the one which must be used when manipulating the glenohumeral joint.

The procedure of manipulation is one of gradually increasing the strength of the stretch, while remaining fully aware of the pressure being applied and the pain being provoked. It should not be a hasty procedure, neither should it be performed too slowly as this will prolong pain unnecessarily. When tearing of structures does occur the physiotherapist must instantly appreciate whether the tear is one 'crack' or a series of minor tears. She instantly decides whether she has gone as far as is necessary or whether she must go on to reach a full range. The decision is a difficult one to make — it is better to underdo the manipulation than to do too much and cause unwarranted pain. Neither medial nor lateral rotation is suitable to be chosen as the technique, the rotary leverage being so great it is difficult to gauge how strongly to proceed: if the contracture is thick and strong the humerus may fracture.

The manipulation should be followed up immediately with repetitive active flexion with the patient lying supine for at least half an hour. This procedure should also be continued hourly at home. At first the patient should concentrate on the gravity-assisted flexion performed supine. This exercise routine performed by the patient should be progressed by the second day to include performing flexion while standing. He should face and stand close to a wall and stretch both arms to a position of maximum flexion. When at the limit of flexion, he should endeavour to lift both arms (with emphasis on the bad arm) up the wall without losing the range of flexion. Flexion should then be exercised actively while the patient lies prone. The patient must be told that if he doesn't exercise properly he will lose his newly acquired range and the fault will be his. Naturally this is not always so but it does produce conscientious exercising.

The patient should be seen the day following the manipulation to check the effectiveness of the home exercising programme in retaining range. Also, if the patient's shoulder is very painful, mobilizing techniques can be used to reduce this pain.

It should be borne in mind that because a patient has a loss of only 15 degrees of flexion it does not mean that he cannot have adhesions. It may prove necessary, even with this seemingly negligible loss of range, to attempt manipulation if firm mobilizing fails to improve range. Manipulation under these circumstances is rarely unsuccessful.

THIRD STAGE

The frozen shoulder has a final stage when the range of movement is restricted but pain free. If the degree of limitation is such that the patient is unable to carry out any functionally important activities, mobilizing can be used strongly in an endeavour to improve the range. The procedure of stretching, say, flexion with grade IV+ movements interspersed with grade IV+ accessory movements at the limit of flexion has been described on page 114. If treatment produces soreness, grade III flexion movements can be used to eliminate it; this has also been described earlier (page 113).

It is unnecessary, and usually unwise, to continue treatment beyond the stage when the active movements are functional. However the patient's pain and movements should be reviewed at intervals. This takes the responsibility regarding any treatment which may be required off the patient's shoulders and puts it fairly and squarely where it should be.

When movements are grossly limited, treatment by passive movement (even MUA) is unlikely to be of any value. It is said that they will regain function with the passage of time.

PAINFULLY STIFF SHOULDER

Many patients are seen who have painful and stiff shoulders which resemble the second stage of a frozen shoulder but who have not had a 'first stage'.

If the range of movement of the glenohumeral joint is limited and very painful when stretched then the treatment is similar to that described earlier ('Second stage, Frozen shoulder'), that is, if treatment of pain fails then the resistance must be treated. Assessment for changes in range and pain must be continued throughout and when a stage of no progress is reached manipulation of the type described above should be considered.

At the initial examination all movements should be assessed for pain and range. The amount by which the pain increases when the movements are stretched is of prime importance. For example, if pain increases rapidly with minor stretching then gentler techniques and larger amplitudes are needed.

Stretching into the quadrant position is the best technique to use initially. As flexion improves, so should all other ranges of movement. However, it may be found that horizontal flexion or the ability to get the hand behind the back do not progress at the same rate. When this is the case, stretching techniques in three directions (quadrant, horizontal flexion and hand behind back) can be used at each treatment session. Whenever stretching techniques are used, accessory movements should also be used at the limit of the particular physiological range being stretched. Accessory or physiological movements should also be used following the stretching but performed more gently and with a large amplitude to reduce treatment soreness. The effectiveness of these latter movements is dramatic.

OSTEOARTHRITIS

It is well documented that osteoarthritis is uncommon in the glenohumeral joint. However, it does occur from time to time and these patients are frequently referred for physiotherapy. In Chapter 5 the treatment of pain was described in detail and it is this treatment which is used for these patients. However, when dealing with the osteoarthritic shoulder the physiotherapist should not change from the postero-anterior accessory movement technique to a flexion or quadrant movement because to do so may cause an exacerbation. In other words, if there is any indication of even minimal crepitus, or if there are arthritic signs in other joints, treatment of the shoulder is more likely to be successful if the accessory movements alone are used. They might need to be grade I or grade II— initially but the aim should be to reach a stage when grade III— (or even III+) movements through the full excursion of the accessory range can be performed without pain.

The physiological movements of abduction, medial or lateral rotation in some degree of glenohumeral abduction, may be used as grade II movements with success.

MINIMAL INTERMITTENT MINOR SHOULDER PAIN

Patients who fit this category usually feel sharp pain when the arm is used unexpectedly, vigorously or in an awkward manner. Examination of the normal movements will prove negative but either the quadrant or the locking position will be found to be positive. When such is the case the more dominant one should be used as the treatment technique.

If the quadrant is being used as the treatment technique then initially the treatment technique should not provoke any pain. It should be performed as very small amplitude grade IV— all around the top of the quadrant position (*Figure 6.41*).

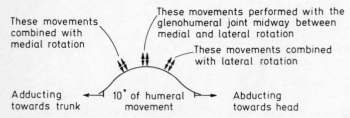

Figure 6.41. — Oscillatory movements, grade IV—, either side of and on top of the quadrant position

As the quadrant becomes less painful a technique whereby the arm rolls back and forth over the quadrant can be used. To do the technique properly the arm is held so that the glenohumeral joint is held medially rotated while the humerus is moved from alongside the head towards and up to the quadrant. Pressure is then exerted against the quadrant and maintained evenly throughout the procedure. As the humerus reaches the top of the quadrant, rotation has been changed to become midway between medial and lateral rotation. Continuing the movement down towards the locking position, the glenohumeral joint is rotated through the neutral mid-position to a position of lateral rotation. At this point of the technique the humerus is pushed towards the head against the quadrant. The arm is then returned to the starting position by being rolled over the quadrant towards the head.

If the locking position is to be treated *(Figure 6.1,* page 66) then gentle oscillatory movements similar to those described for treatment of the quadrant should be used. A scouring type movement as described for *Figure 6.8* (page 76) can be used also.

FRACTURES OF THE HUMERUS

When a patient fractures his humerus the stress causing the fracture also strains the structures supporting the glenohumeral joint. If the fracture is immobilized by a splint which does not encompass the glenohumeral joint, passive movement of the glenohumeral joint can be performed without moving the fracture. There are passive mobilizing techniques which can be applied to the glenohumeral joint which effectively maintain or improve the range of movement available at the glenohumeral joint. This can be achieved even with fractures of the surgical neck of the humeral joint. If the fracture is impacted the dangers are minimal.

These techniques are modifications of those in the preceding text of techniques. The patient's upper arm should be comfortably supported near his trunk and the most important technique would be lateral movement of the head of the humerus as shown in *Figure 6.29* (page 98). The modification necessary would be that, instead of using the hand to produce lateral movement at the glenohumeral joint, the physiotherapist would use one or both of her thumbs high in the axilla on the head of the humerus and the mobilization would be by small amplitude slow oscillatory movements. The second important technique would be postero-anterior movement of the head of the humerus as depicted in *Figure 6.23* (page 92). The third important technique would be produced by longitudinal thumb pressures against the head of the humerus as depicted in *Figure 6.18* (page 87).

Abduction is a most important movement of the glenohumeral joint and should be regained and/or retained as early as possible. Very gentle small amplitude slowly performed oscillatory abduction movements should be performed at the limit of the range. To be sure that there is no movement taking place at the fracture site two rules must be adhered to:

1. The humerus must be supported securely throughout its length.
2. The physiotherapist should firmly imbed her index finger between the lateral border of the acromion process and the head of the humerus so she can freely feel both bones. In this way she can be sure that the humeral head moves in the right proportion as the humerus is abducted.

If the fracture is one which allows the arm to be abducted from the patient's side then modifications of the techniques depicted in *Figures 6.19* (page 88), *6.21* (page 90), *6.27* (page 96) and *6.30* (page 99) may be used whereby the thumb is used directly on the head of the humerus rather than the hand. However, the anteroposterior movement of the head of the humerus in the glenoid cavity as shown in *Figure 6.27* (page 96) is best performed with the physiotherapist's hand over the head of the humerus. This is because it spreads the area of contact.

The techniques referred to above are very effective, not only in assisting range, but also in reducing pain.

ACROMIOCLAVICULAR JOINT PAIN

Pain arising from the acromioclavicular joint is almost invariably felt locally. Rarely does it refer far from the joint but when it does, the referral is usually towards the neck.

The best techniques for treatment of the acromioclavicular joint are those shown in *Figures 6.36, 6.37* and *6.38* (pages 106 and 107). The grades used would be IVs into pain, mixed with grades II and III−.

STERNOCLAVICULAR JOINT

Pain in this joint also causes local pain and the techniques shown in *Figures 6.39* and *6.40* (pages 109 and 110) are most effective. The direction of treatment movement chosen should be one which reproduces the pain and the grades would be the same as for the acromioclavicular joint.

7 Upper Limb

ELBOW JOINT

The elbow joint is complex and consists of the humero-ulnar joint, radiohumeral joint and the superior radio-ulnar joint. Any one of the three can cause pain in the elbow and therefore differential examination of each joint is difficult. It is also necessary to take into consideration that if the elbow is held 5 degrees short of full extension there is an amplitude of abduction/adduction movement. During this abduction/adduction movement the olecranon process swings from side to side in the olecranon fossa, the head of the radius is compressed and distracted from the capitulum and the radius moves cephalad and caudad in the superior radio-ulnar joint.

It is impossible to produce movement in any one of the three joints without producing movement in the others. Therefore, testing movement of one bone on the other must be done by the physiotherapist's fingers and thumbs rather than resorting to gross movements. When movements are tested the accurate site of the pain felt by the patient is a guide in determining which of the joints is at fault.

EXAMINATION

On the whole the elbow joint is inadequately examined by physiotherapists. This accounts, in part, for poor results obtained in physiotherapy treatment of such conditions as tennis elbow.

QUICK TESTS

The patient should be asked to flex fully his elbow actively and then to bounce back and forth at the limit of his flexion range; if he feels pain then the movement should be compared with that on the other side. Extension should be similarly assessed by sharp bouncing movement at the limit of the range. These two quick tests give a useful guide to the extent of elbow joint problems. Following the flexion and extension the patient should be asked to supinate and pronate his forearm as far, as hard and as rapidly as possible.

SPECIAL TESTS

Examination of the physiological movements of flexion, extension, pronation and supination is insufficient to determine the normality or otherwise of this joint. Full use of accessory joint movement must be made if some disturbances are not to be missed. Other authors, and in particular Mennell[1], have discussed the range of lateral accessory movement which is possible when the elbow is held a few degrees from the extended position. This is not the only position in which accessory movements should be assessed. Extension in adduction and extension in abduction are two movements which must be examined when active extension is normal. Similarly, flexion can be examined in both adduction and abduction.

When the elbow is fully extended there is an amplitude of accessory movement from adduction to abduction, which can be represented diagrammatically by a straight line $X_1 Y_1$ (*Figure 7.1*), where X_1 represents adduction and Y_1 represents abduction. If the elbow is now flexed 5 degrees the two positions of adduction and abduction can be represented respectively by another straight line with the limits X_2 and Y_2. The amplitude of this accessory movement is greater in a few degrees of flexion than in the fully extended position.

If the elbow, while firmly held in adduction, is moved from extension through 5 degrees of flexion, that is from X_1 to X_2, it will be felt that the movement is not a straight line but a curve as shown in *Figure 7.1*. The flexion movement in abduction, from Y_1 to Y_2, also follows a slight curve though it is less marked.

Extension/adduction***

The extension/adduction movement is only used in treatment when grade III or IV is required. For the shoulder the quadrant position

[1]   Mennell, John M. (1964). *Joint Pain*. London; Churchill

was described as a point in the abduction to flexion movement. A similar position occurs at the elbow when it is flexed more than 10 degrees from full extension while held in either adduction or abduction. During the first few degrees of flexion in adduction the forearm moves in a plane parallel to the elbow sagittal plane. (The plane of the movement actually slopes slightly away from the sagittal plane as can be seen in *Figure 7.1*). If the flexion is continued, a point is reached where the elbow must be allowed to abduct slightly. This is point X_2 in *Figure 7.1*. Once this point is passed, if the adduction pressure is maintained, the glenohumeral joint will medially rotate. The most important part of the movement is the point near where abduction occurs. The elbow cannot be locked near this roll-over point as can the shoulder (*see* page 66), yet the movement has a similar feel. The two joints are also similar in that when the elbow joint is the source of minor symptoms and its movements appear to be normal, this accessory range may be diminished and painful. In treatment the movement can be scoured in much the same way as was described for the glenohumeral joint (*see* page 75).

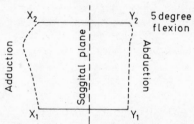

Figure 7.1. – Diagrammatic representation of necessary movement in elbow extension

Starting position

The patient lies far enough from the edge of the couch for his elbow to lie just beyond the edge when his arm is abducted 30 degrees. The physiotherapist, standing by his right shoulder and facing his feet, rests her left forearm in front of, and just medial to, his shoulder. With the fingers of her left hand she supports his elbow from the medial side posteriorly while her thumb extends around the medial epicondylar ridge of the humerus to reach the front of his elbow. The back of her left hand rests against the surface of the couch at its edge. His elbow should be fixed firmly between her hand medially, her fingers and the couch posteriorly, her thumb anteriorly, and her left thigh laterally. This encircling stabilizing grip is essential if the movement is to be performed accurately.

The physiotherapist then grasps the patient's supinated right wrist with her hand, her thumb over the anterior surface and her fingers over the dorsum. The supination is not held strongly at the limit of the range. Once this position is reached she medially rotates his right

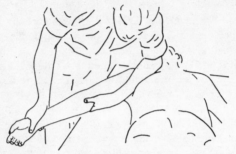

Figure 7.2. – Elbow joint; extension/adduction

glenohumeral joint to stabilize his elbow more easily during adduction; the abduction counterpressure afforded by her left hand is then assisted by the edge of the couch (*Figure 7.2*).

Method

Whenever this movement is used in treatment, the part of the range which is lost or most painful should first be sought. The treatment movement is then usually directed at this particular part of the range in one of two ways. The limitation can be approached by an adduction movement or it can be approached from flexion or extension while the elbow is held adducted. If the line X_1 X_2 represents normal movement, and the dotted line represents abnormal movement found during examination, the direction of the adduction treatment movement is represented by the single-headed arrow and the direction of the flexion/extension treatment movement in adduction is represented by the double-headed arrows (*Figure 7.3a*).

The adduction direction of the treatment movement can be performed as a grade III or IV. If a grade III movement is used, the pressure maintaining adduction is almost completely released to allow the joint to relax to the position almost midway between abduction and adduction before returning to the adduction position. When a grade IV movement is used, the pressure maintaining adduction limits the oscillation to a small amplitude.

The scouring movement is produced by maintaining the adduction pressure while flexing and extending the elbow across the limitation. This type of movement can be further varied if the limitation is very painful by easing the adduction pressure as the pain and limitation are approached. This arc of movement can be performed when extending towards the limitation or flexing towards it. The arc of movement is represented by the arrows showing the direction of the movement in *Figure 7.3b.*

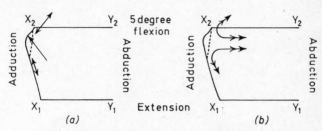

Figure 7.3. – Elbow joint; extension/adduction

Extension/abduction***

Similarly, extension/abduction should be checked from the fully extended position through the first 10 or more degrees of flexion. As with extension/adduction, a point is reached during this range of flexion where the arm must be allowed to adduct if the flexion movement is to be continued. Beyond the point of maximum adduction the arm moves laterally again. This lateral movement will be a lateral rotation of the glenohumeral joint rather than an abduction of the elbow. There is not the same feel of a locking position with this movement as there is with adduction but it is still obvious that the movement from Y_1 to Y_2 in *Figure 7.1* is not a straight line but is slightly curved. Any loss of the smooth contour of this curve can be appreciated and can be treated by movement into this position.

Starting position

The starting position is similar to that described for extension/adduction with the exception of the physiotherapist's grip of the patient's wrist. She holds his supinated wrist from the medial side with her fingers spreading over the back of his wrist and her thumb over the front. If his glenohumeral joint is slightly laterally rotated the abduction movement can be directed against her thigh which then acts as the fulcrum (*Figure 7.4*).

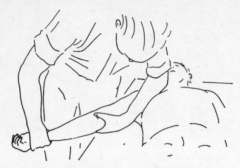

Figure 7.4. – Elbow joint; extension/abduction

Method

Movements are performed in the same way as in extension/adduction. Flexion/extension movements or circular movements can be performed while maintaining an abduction pressure in much the same way as one would scour a hollow. An abduction movement can be directed at the limitation of the painful part of the range from midway between abduction or adduction using grade III or IV movements. For each method the patient's elbow must be firmly fixed by the physiotherapist's hand against a very firm fulcrum.

The above are examples of extension/abduction and extension/adduction being used as examination procedures and yet also being used for treatment.

Flexion/abduction and flexion/adduction

These two movements should also be used as special tests for the elbow. They are described on pages 132 and 134. They too, can be used for examination and treatment. When used for examination purposes a grade IV to grade IV+ is used.

Tables 7.1, 7.2 and 7.3 provide the pattern of examination for each of the three joints which comprise the elbow. As mentioned above the site of pain produced by any of the test movements will help to indicate which joint is involved. It is also useful to have a 'composite table' (Table 7.4) as there is considerable overlap in the test movements used for each of the individual joints.

Table 7.1
Humero-ulnar Joint: Objective Examination

[The routine examination of this joint must also include examination of the superior radio-ulnar (R/U) joint as supinator/pronator torsion is possible at the humero-ulnar joint]

Observation

Active movements

Acitve quick tests (+cervical)

Routinely

F, E, Sup and Pron in F and E

Note range, pain, repeated and rapid

As applicable

Speed of test movements

Specific movements which aggravate

The injuring movement

Movements under load

Thoracic outlet tests

Muscle power

Static tests

Muscles in 'plan' including clenching fist in different positions of elbow

Other joints in 'plan'

Passive movements

Physiological movements

Routinely

F, E, Sup and Pron in F and E

Note range, pain, resistance, spasm and behaviour

As applicable

E/Ab, E/Ad, F/Ab, F/Ad, Ab and Ad in 5 degrees F

Accessory movements

As applicable

1. →→ , ←← , ←→→ caudad on olecranon and coronoid
2. ←→→ ceph and caud at 90 degrees, i.e.

   (*a*) in line with ulna

   (*b*) in line with humerus in different angles between full F and E

Note range, pain, resistance, spasm and behaviour

Palpation

Temperature

Swelling and wasting

Altered sensation

Relevant tenderness (ulnar nerve hypersensitivity)

Check case records etc.

HIGHLIGHT MAIN FINDINGS WITH ASTERISKS

After treatment

TECHNIQUES

Extension

Extension is commonly used in grades II and III— but when the joint is only mildly painful grades III and IV may be used.

GRADE II***

Starting position

The physiotherapist stands by the patient's right hip, facing his head, and rests her right knee on the couch. With her left hand she supports laterally around his right arm just above his elbow with her thumb anteriorly and her fingers posteriorly. She grasps the palm of his

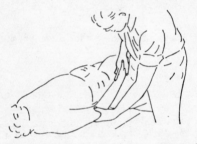

Figure 7.5. – Elbow joint; extension, grade II

supinated hand with her right hand; her thumb reaches between his thumb and index finger to the back of his hand and her medial three fingers reach around the hypothenar eminence to the back of his hand. Her index finger points proximally over the anterior aspect of his wrist. She moves close to his elbow and uses her thigh to provide the stop at the required angle (*Figure 7.5*).

Method

The oscillatory movement is performed entirely by the physiotherapist's right arm while her left hand acts as a comfortable support around the patient's elbow. With her grasp of his right wrist she endeavours to encourage relaxation in this area and throughout the arm. The amplitude of movement is approximately 20–30 degrees.

GRADE III

If grade III movements are used when the elbow has a limited range of extension the starting position is identical with that described for grade II. However, if the range is nearly full a different starting position is required.

*Starting position***

The patient lies with his arm abducted approximately 15 degrees so that his wrist is clear of the edge of the couch. The physiotherapist stands by his right shoulder, facing his feet, and supports under his elbow from the medial side with her left hand while holding his shoulder down with her left forearm. With her right hand she grasps his supinated wrist laterally, her thenar eminence and thumb pointing distally across the front of his wrist and her fingers across the back of his wrist and hand (*Figure 7.6a*).

Method

The oscillation is done entirely by the physiotherapist's right hand, and the patient's right hand is stabilized by her grasp of his wrist. The amplitude of elbow movement is approximately 20–30 degrees.

*Alternative starting position****

There is another technique which sometimes provides a better feeling of the last 30 degrees of extension and it is a technique which allows some patients to relax more easily.

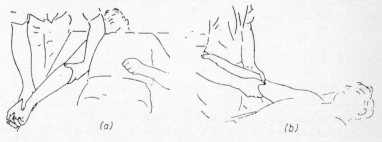

(a)   *(b)*

Figure 7.6. – Elbow joint; extension, grade III

The physiotherapist stands by the patient's right hip, facing his head. She lifts his right arm and holds his hand against her right side. She holds around his elbow with both hands, her thumbs holding anterior to the joint and her fingers overlapping posteriorly (*Figure 7.6b*).

Alternative method

The oscillation is produced by raising and lowering the patient's elbow 4 or 5 inches while his wrist is stabilized. The treatment may be assisted by applying either compression or slight distraction to his elbow by her grasp of his wrist. Adduction or abduction can also be added to the extension movement by increasing the pressure in either direction by her left or right hand.

GRADE IV

This movement should never be performed more strongly than as a grade IV—.

Starting position***

The starting position is identical with that described for *Figure 7.6a* except that the physiotherapist's hand and knee should be the fulcrum for the movement rather than the couch. This position enables a more perceptive feel of the strength of the oscillation.

Flexion

Passive movement in this direction is a very useful treatment procedure, particularly with grade III or IV.

GRADE II**

Starting position

The physiotherapist stands by the patient's right shoulder facing his feet and supports under his right elbow from the medial side with her left forearm crossing his right upper arm. With her right hand she grasps his supinated wrist from the lateral side with her fingers across the back of his hand, and her thumb between his thumb and index finger into his palm. To provide the stop for the flexion movement, she flexes his elbow to the required position and then raises her left fore-arm until it is in firm contact with the front of his right wrist (*Figure 7.7*).

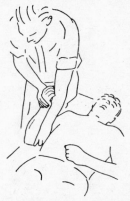

Figure 7.7. – Elbow joint; flexion, grade II

Method

The oscillatory movement, performed by the physiotherapist's right arm, is taken back and forth through 20–30 degrees up to the stop provided by her left forearm. As the range improves her left forearm can be lowered.

GRADES III AND IV**

When the range of flexion is limited and grades III and IV are required a similar starting position to that adopted for grade II is used. However, if the movement is almost full range a different starting position is required.

Starting position

The physiotherapist stands by the patient's right side, distal to his elbow, facing his head. With her left hand she supports his right upper arm just above the elbow. She flexes and supinates his elbow holding the back of his hand with her right hand, her thumb passing through the first interosseous space, her medial three fingers spreading medially around the fifth metacarpal and her index finger extending distally along the back of his hand (*Figure 7.8*).

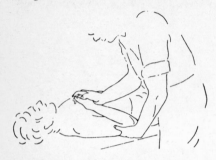

*Figure 7.8. – Elbow joint; flexion,
grades III and IV*

Method

The oscillation is produced entirely by moving the patient's right arm while her left hand acts as a support under his elbow. Grade III movements are large with amplitudes of between 10 and 30 degrees reaching the limit of the flexion range, and grade IV movements are small amplitude oscillations of 3 or 4 degrees.

Flexion with accessory movement

Frequently a joint exhibiting minimal symptoms may have a full range of flexion. It is inadequate under these circumstances to test flexion only as a straight movement. There are three ways the movement can be varied and during examination these should be tested with grade IV type movements before determining that flexion is a painless full range. These movements are flexion/adduction, flexion/abduction and flexion with distraction. When employed in treatment they are used only in grades III or IV.

Flexion/adduction***

Starting position

The physiotherapist stands by the patient's right hip, facing his head, and fully pronates his forearm. She holds his fully pronated wrist with her left hand, her fingers over the back of his wrist and her thenar eminence and thumb over the front. She grasps firmly from the medial side around his upper arm at the junction of the middle and lower thirds in such a way as to hold his upper arm laterally rotated. The slack in soft tissue must be taken up fully. Both forearms are then directed opposite each other (*Figure 7.9*).

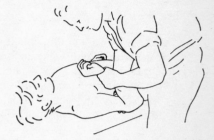

Figure 7.9. – Elbow joint; flexion/ adduction

Method

The flexion/adduction movement is performed entirely by the physiotherapist's left arm while she prevents any medial rotation of the glenohumeral joint with her firm grasp of his upper arm. If medial rotation is not prevented, the adduction strain at his elbow will be lost. The treatment movement can be performed as large amplitude oscillations through 10–15 degrees (grade III) or as small oscillatory movements through 3 or 4 degrees (grade IV).

Flexion/abduction***

Starting position

The physiotherapist stands by the patient's right hip, facing his head, while supporting under his upper arm with her left hand and flexing his elbow with her right hand. With her left hand she grasps his upper

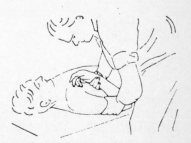

Figure 7.10. – Elbow joint; flexion/abduction

arm at the junction of the middle and lower thirds in such a way as to prevent lateral rotation of the glenohumeral joint. With her right hand she grasps his supinated wrist from the medial side, her fingers spreading across the front of his wrist and her thumb across the back (*Figure 7.10*).

Method

She flexes his elbow and displaces it laterally with an abduction movement at the elbow joint, while applying an equal counterpressure with her left hand, preventing any lateral rotation of the glenohumeral joint. If this counterpressure is unsuccessful, the sideways movement of the patient's wrist will consist of lateral rotation of the glenohumeral joint without any abduction at the elbow.

Flexion with longitudinal caudad movement**

This is the least useful of the three accessory movements associated with flexion.

Starting position

The physiotherapist stands by the patient's right hip, facing his head. She flexes his elbow with her right hand, grasping around the medial aspect of his supinated wrist, her fingers spreading across the front and

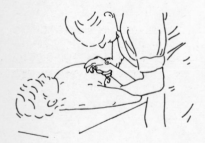

Figure 7.11. – Elbow joint; flexion with longitudinal movement caudad in full elbow flexion

her thumb across the back. When his elbow reaches 90 degrees of flexion she places her supinated left forearm just proximal to her wrist, in the crook of his elbow. Elbow flexion is continued until her left wrist is firmly squeezed between his forearm and upper arm (*Figure 7.11*).

Method

The movement consists of small oscillations produced by the physiotherapist's right arm. Care is needed to maintain her wedged arm in a
constant proximity to the patient's elbow because the tendency will be
for it to be squeezed out. A wrong degree of supination forming the
wedge will make the position very uncomfortable for the patient.

Longitudinal caudad movement (90 degrees flexion)*

This movement should be tested when joint signs are minimal. It is a
mobilization used in the treatment of stiff elbows.

Starting position

The physiotherapist stands by the patient's right elbow, facing his left
knee, and flexes his right elbow to a right-angle. She supports the back
of his supinated right wrist by grasping around his medial metacarpals

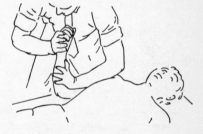

*Figure 7.12. – Elbow joint;
longitudinal movement caudad
(90 degrees flexion)*

with her fingers and through the first interosseous space with her
thumb while maintaining his wrist in a neutral position. She places the
heel of her left hand over the anterior aspect of his upper forearm with
her fingers spreading distally down the front of his forearm. Her left
thumb spreads laterally around his forearm and her three medial
fingers spread medially (*Figure 7.12*).

Method

The slack of scapulothoracic depression must be taken up before
alternating pressures are applied against the forearm to produce the
distraction movement. There is very little movement in this direction

and it is almost impossible to feel any localized accessory movement. The movement can be combined with minimal elbow flexion movement or the physiotherapist can carry the patient's hand with the movement, maintaining a constant elbow angle.

Sometimes distraction is produced better by thumb pressure against the anterior surface of the ulna.

Alternative starting position**

The physiotherapist stands by the patient's right hip, facing his head. His arm is flexed and supported against her right hip anteriorly. She then grasps his forearm near the elbow, placing the pads of her thumbs against the coronoid process. The fingers of her right hand spread

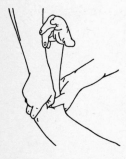

Figure 7.13. — Elbow joint; longitudinal movement caudad (90 degrees flexion), alternative position

medially around his forearm and those of her left hand spread laterally. She should position her index fingers so that their lateral margins are in contact with the distal margin of the medial and lateral epicondyles (*Figure 7.13*).

Alternative method

The movement is produced by the arms acting through the pads of the thumbs while counterpressure is exerted through the index fingers against the epicondyles. The pressure must not be created by the thumb flexors as the movement then becomes uncomfortable for the patient and all feeling of movement is lost.

Distraction can be performed in different positions of elbow flexion, and during treatment it may be necessary to carry out the distraction movement in more than one position of elbow flexion.

SUPERIOR RADIO-ULNAR JOINT

As well as supination and pronation, the superior radio-ulnar joint has passive accessory movements of the head of the radius on the ulna. These are postero-anterior and anteroposterior movements, which can be performed with the forearm in any degree of elbow supination or pronation, flexion or extension. Longitudinal movements cephalad and caudad are the two remaining accessory movements, though they have limited practical application. All of these movements can be performed with or without compression of the head of the radius against the ulna (Table 7.2).

Table 7.2
Superior Radio-ulnar Joint: Objective Examination

[The routine examination of this joint must also include examination of the elbow joint]

Observation

Active movements
　　As described for the elbow joint

Static tests

Other joints in 'plan'

Passive movements
Physiological movements
　　As for elbow joint
Accessory movements
　　Routinely
　　　　1. Ab and Ad of elbow in 5 degrees F
　　　　2. ←•→ cephalad and caudad in different angles of elbow F and E and different angles of Sup and Pron (using wrist deviations)
　　　　3. ↕ and ↕ , each from full pronation to full supination
　　　　4. Supination/pronation under compression

Palpation

Check case records etc.

HIGHLIGHT MAIN FINDINGS WITH ASTERISKS

After treatment

Supination***

As the techniques for grades I to IV are similar, whether the range is restricted or not, the movement will only be described as a grade II and IV+ movement in a full range joint.

Starting position

The physiotherapist stands by the patient's right side beyond his flexed elbow, facing his head, and supports under his elbow with her left hand. With her right hand she grasps his supinated wrist from the medial side, her fingers spreading across the front of his wrist and carpus and her thumb across the back (*Figure 7.14*).

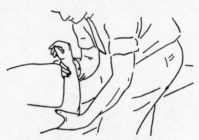

Figure 7.14. – Superior radio-ulnar joint;
supination grades I–IV

Method

A grade II movement requires a very flicky action by the physiotherapist's right hand. It is performed from midway between supination and pronation to full supination. The supination is produced by a combined action of the physiotherapist's own supination with flexion of her wrist and fingers. During the movement the patient's wrist must be stabilized to prevent flapping.

When grades III and IV are performed, the physiotherapist must support the patient's elbow medially to prevent glenohumeral adduction, or alternatively, she must begin the movement with the patient's elbow adducted against his side.

For stronger grades of movement a different starting position is adopted which places the physiotherapist in a more economical working position.

GRADE IV+**

Starting position

The physiotherapist stands by the patient's flexed right elbow and holds the distal end of his fully supinated radius and ulna in her left and right hands respectively holding far enough distally to stabilize the

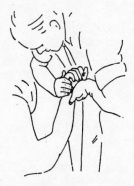

Figure 7.15. – Superior radio-ulnar joint; supination grade IV+

hand. She fully supinates her left forearm and holds the distal end of his radius posteriorly with the lateral surface of the distal phalanx of her index finger and anteriorly with the pad of her thumb. With her right hand she holds the distal end of the ulna, her thumb and thenar eminence pointing distally over the back of his wrist and her fingers holding anteriorly. Her forearms are directed opposite each other at right angles to the coronal plane of the fully supinated wrist (*Figure 7.15*).

Method

Keeping her forearm in the same line, she pronates his forearm 2 or 3 degrees by pulling on his radius and ulna and then returns it to the fully supinated position. Her action is one of alternately easing her hands apart and pushing them back together again. Repetition of this action produces the oscillatory supination. The amplitude is small (4 or 5 degrees) and if the joint range is limited she merely turns her body towards the right to change the direction of her forearms.

Pronation***

Starting position

The physiotherapist stands by the patient's right hip facing his head, supporting under his flexed elbow with her right hand so that her fingers can reach the lateral surface. With her left hand she grasps his

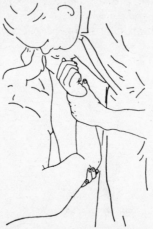

Figure 7.16. – Superior radio-ulnar joint; pronation

pronated forearm distally, her fingers extending across the dorsum of his wrist and hand to reach the carpus and her thumb extending around the anterior surface. This position is necessary to stabilize the wrist during the pronation movements (*Figure 7.16*).

Method

The physiotherapist performs the rotary movement by slight gleno-humeral flexion combined with slight extension of the left shoulder and elbow to move her arm forward. This action is combined with full flexion of her wrist and fingers to produce the pronation. With her right hand she stabilizes his upper arm, preventing abduction of his shoulder.

A more efficient position for grade IV+ movements can be used.

GRADE IV+**

Starting position

The physiotherapist stands by the patient's elbow, facing across his body. His elbow is flexed to 90 degrees and pronated. She grasps the distal end of his radius and ulna with her left and right hands respectively. She places the thenar eminence of her left hand against the dorsal surface of the radius with her thumb extending distally across the back of his wrist while her fingers grasp anteriorly around his radius. With her right hand fully supinated she grasps around the distal

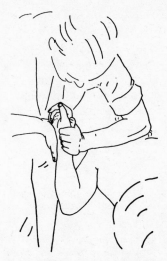

*Figure 7.17. – Superior radio-ulnar
joint; pronation, grade IV+*

end of his ulna, the heel of her hand and her thumb pointing proximally against the anterior surface of the ulna and her fingers grasping around the ulna to reach the posterior surface. She directs her forearms opposite each other (*Figure 7.17*).

Method

The oscillatory pronation is produced by the same method as that described for supination.

Anteroposterior movement

Although the range of movement is greatest when the forearm is midway between pronation and supination, the technique is more commonly used in either the fully supinated or pronated position. It is used most when loss of range is more important to the patient than his pain, but it is also important when minor symptoms arise from the joint when the pain can be elicited by this technique. The treatment usually involves grade III or IV movements and it is described here in a position of approximately 30 degrees elbow flexion and full supination and pronation.

IN SUPINATION***

Starting position

The physiotherapist stands by the patient's right side beyond his slightly flexed right elbow, facing his head. She supports the back of his supinated forearm against her right side and places the pads of her thumbs over the anterior surface of the head of the radius. She should

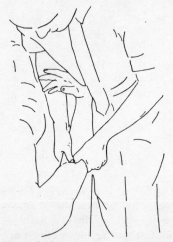

Figure 7.18. — Superior radio-ulnar joint;
anteroposterior movement in supination

gradually apply pressure with her thumbs so they sink into the relaxed muscle tissue to contact the head of the radius. The fingers of her left and right hands spread over the lateral and medial surfaces of the upper end of the forearm (*Figure 7.18*).

Method

The oscillations are produced by the physiotherapist's arms and the pressure is transmitted through her thumbs, which act as springs. The pressure required for the mobilization must not be produced by the thumb flexor muscles.

IN PRONATION

Starting position

The starting position is similar to that described above for supination (*Figure 7.18*) except that the physiotherapist holds the patient's pronated right wrist around its lateral border with her right hand, her thumb crosses the back of his wrist and her fingers cross the front. It is

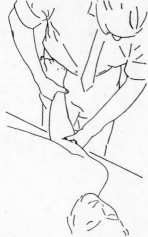

Figure 7.19. – Superior radio-ulnar joint;
anteroposterior movement in pronation

necessary to hold his forearm in pronation because the anteroposterior pressure tends to produce supination. She supports his forearm against her side and places her left thumb against the head of the radius and her fingers around the lateral surface of the forearm (*Figure 7.19*).

Method

The mobilization is performed by the physiotherapist's left arm through the stable thumb while maintaining the pronation with her right hand.

Postero-anterior movement

This movement has a similar application in treatment to the antero-posterior movement and therefore grade III and IV movements are the ones commonly used. Also it can be performed in varying degrees of elbow flexion extension, supination or pronation. Postero-anterior movement will be described with the elbow in approximately 30 degrees of flexion at the limits of both supination and pronation.

IN SUPINATION***

Starting position

The physiotherapist stands by the patient's right side beyond his slightly flexed elbow, facing his head, and holds his supinated wrist from the medial side with her right hand. She places her thumb across the front of his wrist and her fingers across the back. The pad of her left thumb, pointing distally, is placed against the dorsal surface of the

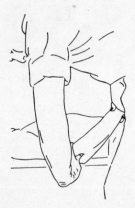

*Figure 7.20. – Superior radio-ulnar joint;
postero-anterior movement in supination*

head of the radius. To provide a counterpressure for the movement, her fingers are placed against the front of the distal end of the upper arm. Because this movement tends to produce pronation it is necessary to stabilize the patient's wrist in supination (*Figure 7.20*).

Method

The physiotherapist produces the movement by small adduction movements of her left shoulder combined with slight forearm supination to exert pressure against the head of the radius with her left thumb. If the pressure is produced by the flexors of the thumb, the feel of the movement will be lost and the pressure will be uncomfortable to both patient and operator.

IN PRONATION***

Starting position

The same starting position and method are adopted as have been described for postero-anterior movement in supination (*Figure 7.20*) except that the wrist is held with the forearm pronated.

Longitudinal movement caudad*

This movement can, like the other accessory movements, be performed with the elbow in any degree of flexion, extension, supination or pronation. However, if maximum range of movement in the normal joint is required the forearm should be positioned midway between flexion and extension and also midway between supination and pronation. The movement will be described in this position but other positions can be used. The position used in treatment is commonly the one found to be most restricted or most painful.

Starting position

The physiotherapist stands by the patient's right side just beyond his elbow and rests his right forearm against her right side. She holds across the front of his upper arm, proximal to his elbow, with her left hand, her fingers spreading laterally and her thumb medially. Her main point of contact against his upper arm is the web of her first interosseous space. With her right hand she grasps the anterior surface of his supinated carpus. Her thumb grasps around the radial surface proximal to the base of the fifth metacarpal. The middle finger and thumb must reach as far as possible around the posterior surface of the carpus. Her right forearm must then be brought into the same line as the patient's forearm (*Figure 7.21*).

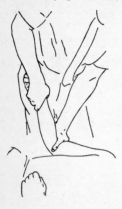

Figure 7.21. – Superior radio-ulnar joint; longitudinal movement caudad

Method

When this technique is used as a grade IV movement, which is its most common use, the slack in soft tissue must first be taken up. As the physiotherapist pulls with her right hand her left hand must sink into the patient's flexor muscle tissue to hold his upper arm firmly. Slack must also be taken up at the wrist. Small oscillatory longitudinal movements can then be performed by a pulling action with her right arm counteracted by an equal and opposite pressure through her left hand. Ulnar deviation should also be performed in time with the pulling action.

Longitudinal movement cephalad*

This movement is mainly used as a grade IV movement in positions between 90 degrees flexion and full flexion. The technique will be described with the patient's forearm midway between supination and pronation in 90 degrees of flexion.

Starting position

The physiotherapist stands by the patient's right side beyond his flexed elbow facing his head and grasps his right hand in hers as if shaking hands. She then extends her right wrist, and his, and supports under the distal end of his right upper arm with her left hand. She crouches over his hand and supports her right hand against her right hip (*Figure 7.22*).

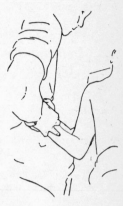

Figure 7.22. – Superior radio-ulnar joint; longitudinal movement cephalad

Method

There is no slack to be taken up with this movement and the small oscillations are produced by pressure through the physiotherapist's wrist along the line of the shaft of the radius together with radial deviation of the wrist joint.

RADIOHUMERAL JOINT

Symptoms do not commonly arise from this joint unless it has been involved in trauma or unless there is some disorder of the elbow or superior radio-ulnar joint.

The main technique used in examining this joint (Table 7.3) is to apply a compressive force through the patient's hand so as to compress the head of the radius against the capitulum. The technique is shown in *Figure 7.22* above, with the elbow in approximately 90 degrees of flexion. To localize the movement as much as possible to the radio-humeral joint the pressure should be transmitted through the patient's thenar eminence with the wrist deviated radially directing the force through the radius. The compression technique should be performed through as large a range of elbow flexion to extension range as is possible.

If the technique described above does not produce any symptoms then a supination to pronation oscillatory movement should be added to the compressing of the head of the radius against the humerus. Again, this should be performed in many positions of elbow flexion and extension.

Table 7.3
Radiohumeral Joint: Objective Examination

[The routine examination of this joint must include examination of other joints making up the elbow]

Observation

Active movements
      Active quick tests (+cervical)
    Routinely
      F, E; Sup and Pron in F and E
      Note range, pain, repeated and rapid
    As applicable
      Speed of test movements
      Specific movements which aggravate
      The injuring movement
      Movements under load
      Thoracic outlet tests
      Muscle power

Static tests
    Muscles in 'plan' including clenching fist in different positions

Other joints in 'plan'

Passive movements
    Routinely
    1. F, E; Sup and Pron in F and E
    2. ←→ ceph and caud (by wrist deviations) in different angles of elbow full F to full E
    3. Distraction in 90 degrees elbow F
    4. While radiohumeral (R/H) joint compressed and in 90 degrees F to E and Sup to Pron do ↕ and ↕

    Note range, pain, resistance, spasm and behaviour

Palpation

Check case records etc.

HIGHLIGHT MAIN FINDINGS WITH ASTERISKS

After treatment

TREATMENT

When pain is felt by the patient in a vague area around the elbow joint it is very difficult to determine which of the three joints is the primary one at fault. During examination, the accessory movements performed at the limit of the various ranges may provide the answer. In many circumstances elbow extension or extension in conjunction with abduction or adduction will provide the most comparable sign and therefore these are the most commonly used techniques in treatment. However, if an accessory movement at the limit of a physiological range is a good 'comparable sign' then it would be the first technique used.

The elbow, whether being treated for pain or stiffness, is a joint which is extremely easily overtreated at any one session. Therefore, if the physiological movement of extension is used to treat pain it is vital that the patient's arm be completely relaxed during treatment, and the technique should be completely free of even the most minor feeling of discomfort. The technique shown in *Figure 7.6b* (page 129) is commonly the best position in which to use grades II and III— extension. This is because the joint is completely surrounded and supported by both hands while the forearm and hand can be comfortably surrounded and supported by the physiotherapist's forearm and trunk.

If the patient's symptoms are comparatively mild, and gentle grade IV extension movements are contemplated as treatment techniques, initially movements should be slower than those usually used and the amount of pain provoked by the treatment should be minimal. If this care is not taken the patient will almost certainly have an exacerbation.

Tennis elbow

If the term tennis elbow is used accurately, then passive movements of the joints will be full range and painless. Under these circumstances passive movement techniques have no place in treatment. (In the author's experience, Mill's manipulation, when used effectively, produces a good result because it manipulates the joint and not because it has stretched the tenomuscular junction at the lateral epicondyle.)

The term tennis elbow in the majority of cases is used loosely and careful examination will reveal that there is a joint component to the symptoms as well as the tenomuscular component. When minor joint signs are present they should be used as the passive movement treatment techniques. Initially, the joint signs alone should be treated until a clear picture of the pattern of progress can be predicted. It may then be necessary to treat the tenomuscular component while continuing with the joint treatment. However, on many occasions, the tenomuscular component recovers spontaneously when joint movement recovers.

Most tennis elbows which have become chronic will have a joint component as part of the comparable joint signs.

Joint stiffness

The long-held view that stretching the elbow is likely to cause a myositis ossificans is taking a long time to die. When a patient has a stiff and painful joint the physiotherapist should treat the pain first so that she has a clear picture of its behaviour and irritability. Once this is known and treatment is directed towards stretching the elbow in any direction provided progression of the strength of the technique used does not unfavourably alter the pattern of the pain, the stretching techniques are completely safe. As has been indicated earlier the stretching techniques would consist of three elements:

1. A physiological movement is selected and grade IV or IV– stretching can be applied provided pain is minimal.
2. The joint is now supported at the limit of the range being stretched and accessory movements (for example *Figure 7.13*, page 136) are also performed as grade IV movements.
3. Either interspersed between the physiological movements and the accessory movements, or at the completion of the treatment session, gradeII+ (or III– if not painful) are used through as large a range as is possible.

Chronic minor joint pain

When a patient has pain in the elbow which is minor and the condition has existed without change for a long time then the techniques used will be the 'comparable signs' found at examination. After the first examination and treatment, if the disorder is found to be not irritable, then subsequent treatments must be performed as grade IV or IV+ movements interspersed with grade III and III+ movements.

If the patient has a seemingly full range of movement and the comparable signs are found to be very close to the limit of the range then the two most commonly used techniques are extension/adduction while the elbow is positioned approximately 5 degrees short of full extension, or extension/abduction in the same degree of elbow flexion. These techniques, when used at the right time on the right patient, are dramatic in their relief of pain.

GENERAL EXAMINATION OF THE ELBOW JOINT

Movements of the three joints which combine to form the elbow do not occur in isolation. It is therefore difficult at times to determine whether pain felt on stretching supination, for example, is in fact

Table 7.4
Composite Elbow Joint: Objective Examination

Observation

Active movements
    Active quick tests
    Routinely
    F, E; Bouncing F and E in full pronation and supination

Static tests

Other joints in 'plan'

Passive movements
    Routinely
    F, E Sup and Pron as IV– to IV+ to III++
    Differentiating as required
    1. F and E as IV+ at limit of range
        (*a*) F/Ab, F/Ad, E/Ab, E/Ad, Ab/Ad in 5 degrees F
        (*b*) ◄◄► (in line with humerus) ceph and caud
            (*i*) on radius (R/H joint or superior R/U joint)
               add superior R/U compression to differentiate between R/H and superior R/U
            (*ii*) on ulna (humero-ulnar joint)
        (*c*) ◄◄► (in line with radius) ceph and caud
            (*i*) on radius (R/H or superior R/U joint)
               add superior R/U compression to differentiate between R/H and superior R/U
            (*ii*) on ulna (humero-ulnar joint)
    2. Sup and Pron as IV+ at limit of range
        (*a*) ↕ , ↑ on head of radius (superior R/U or R/H joint)
        add compression of superior R/U joint to differentiate between radiohumeral and superior R/U joint
        (*b*) ↕ , ↑ on ulna (humero-ulnar joint)
    3. Other differentiating tests
        (*a*) ↕ , ↘ , ↗ , ↕ , ↖ , ↗ on head of radius in different positions of elbow F and E
        (*b*) →► ◄◄ on olecranon and coronoid

Palpation

Check case records etc.

HIGHLIGHT MAIN FINDINGS WITH ASTERISKS

After treatment

arising from the superior radio-ulnar joint. This is because if supination is stretched, the humero-ulnar joint undergoes a degree of torsion and the head of the radius spins and slides under the capitulum. Table 7.4 lists the test movements performed, and shows how supination, for example, can be performed in a way to differentiate between the components of the movement.

INFERIOR RADIO-ULNAR JOINT

The passive movements which can be produced at the inferior radio-ulnar joint are supination, pronation, postero-anterior (PA) and antero-posterior (AP) movements of the ulna on the radius. The last two movements can be produced with the inferior radio-ulnar joint positioned anywhere from the limit of pronation to the limit of supination. The largest amplitude of the movement is when the inferior radio-ulnar joint is positioned midway between full pronation and supination. The PA and AP movements are referred to as movements of the ulna on the radius because it is easier to stabilize the comparatively large distal end of the radius and produce the movement by pushing the distal end of the ulna.

The next movement possible at the radio-ulnar joint, either actively or passively, is described as being longitudinal movement of the radius on the ulna either cephalad or caudad. The reasons for presenting the movement as being that of the radius on the ulna are: first, the ulna is relatively more stable and second, one of the best ways of producing this movement is to carry out ulnar deviation of the hand, which pulls the radius in a caudad direction. Cephalad longitudinal movement of the radius on the ulna is produced by radial deviation of the wrist.

One last movement which can be produced passively at the inferior radio-ulnar joint consists of compression, where the radius and ulna are squeezed together, and distraction, when the distal ends of the radius and ulna are separated.

EXAMINATION

During the examination of the inferior radio-ulnar joint when the forearm is supinated or pronated strongly and the patient feels pain in the vicinity of the inferior radio-ulnar joint it is commonly erroneously assumed that the pain is arising from that joint. When it is realized that supination and pronation can also be produced at the wrist joint it is easy to see how this error is made.

QUICK TESTS

These tests consist of asking the patient to flick his forearm through a large amplitude, firstly striking the limit of supination four or five times and then repeating the technique for pronation.

SPECIAL TESTS

There are two important special tests for the inferior radio-ulnar joint. The first is performed when the inferior radio-ulnar joint is stretched to

Table 7.5
Inferior Radio-ulnar Joint: Objective Examination

[The routine examination of this joint must also include examination of the wrist, as supination and pronation also occur as accessory movements of the wrist joint]

Observation

Active movements
     Active quick tests
    Routinely
       Wrist F, E, Ab, Ad, supination, pronation
       Note range, pain, repeated and rapid

Static tests

Other joints in 'plan'

Passive movements
Physiological movements
    Routinely
       Sup and Pron
       Note range, pain, resistance, spasm and behaviour
Accessory movements
    As applicable
    1. ↕ ↕
      (*a*) in neutral (also ↕)
      (*b*) at limit of pronation
      (*c*) at limit of supination
    2. Sup/Pron with compression as c.f. distraction
    3. Sup and Pron differentiating
      Note range, pain, resistance, spasm and behaviour

Palpation

Check records etc.

HIGHLIGHT MAIN FINDINGS WITH ASTERISKS

After treatment

the limit of, say, supination. While the joint is held in this position an extra anteroposterior movement should be exerted against the anterior surface of the ulna and after assessing pain with this movement a postero-anterior movement should be applied from the posterior surface of the ulna. The same anteroposterior and postero-anterior movements should be performed with the ulna moving on the radius at the limit of pronation.

The second special test is to compress strongly the radius against the ulna and at the same time rock the radius and ulna back and forth against each other. This technique is shown in *Figure 7.24* (page 155).

Table 7.5 lists the full passive movement examination.

TECHNIQUES

Postero-anterior and anteroposterior movements***

Starting position

The physiotherapist stands by the patient's right side, just beyond his flexed elbow, facing his left shoulder. She holds his forearm, midway between supination and pronation, between the thumb and index finger of each hand. The distal end of his radius is held in her left hand between the thumb on the posterior surface and the flexed index finger on the anterior surface. If all her fingers are flexed they can be used to add lateral support to the index finger which makes the main point of contact. With her right hand she holds the distal end of his ulna with an identical grip (*Figure 7.23*).

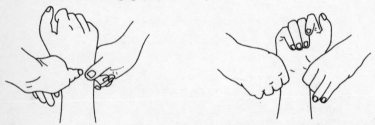

Figure 7.23. – Inferior radio-ulnar joint; postero-anterior and anteroposterior movements

Method

A postero-anterior movement of the radius on the ulna is produced by pressure against the anterior surface of the ulna with the physiotherapist's right index finger and an equal and opposite pressure against the posterior surface of the head of the radius with her left thumb. Obviously, an anteroposterior movement of the head of the radius on the ulna would be produced by an opposite action.

If either of these movements needs to be performed strongly at the limit of its range, the physiotherapist should grasp the radius and ulna more firmly between the thenar eminence, rather than just the thumb, and the respective fingers. The oscillation is then produced by a pushing and pulling action of the arms.

Compression**

Starting position

The physiotherapist kneels by the patient's right side beyond his flexed elbow and grasps his right hand in her two hands. Her thumb and thenar eminence, pointing towards his fingers, cover the posterior surface of his wrist, meeting in the mid line. Her fingers reach around to meet anteriorly in the mid line. The heel of her left hand cups around the lateral surface of the distal end of his radius while the heel of her right hand cups around his ulna. Both arms are directed opposite to each other at right angles to his forearm (*Figure 7.24*).

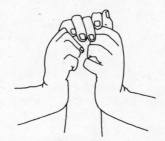

*Figure 7.24. – Inferior radio-ulnar joint;
compression*

Method

Supination and pronation are produced by a twisting in opposite directions of the heels of the physiotherapist's hands pivoting around her stationary fingers and thumbs. Pronation of the patient's forearm is produced by pronation of her left forearm and supination of her right forearm so that the heels of her hands move away from each other. Supination is produced by supination of her left forearm combined with pronation of her right. A back and forth rocking movement between supination and pronation is continued while the compression is maintained between her two arms.

Longitudinal movement cephalad*

Starting position and method

The technique is almost identical with that shown in *Figure 7.22* (page 147) but emphasis must be placed on the exact position of the patient's hand and the direction of the pressure applied by the physiotherapist's hand. The patient's hand must be tilted towards radial deviation and the physiotherapist should apply her main contact through the base of the patient's thenar eminence so that the pressure is in a straight line with the shaft of the radius.

Longitudinal movement caudad*

Starting position and method

This is identical with that shown in *Figure 7.21* (page 146) but with one special qualification. The physiotherapist must grasp around the patient's hand immediately adjacent to the base of the first metacarpal and the pisiform bone. During the movement longitudinally the patient's wrist should be deviated towards the ulnar side.

It is important to realize that during radial deviation of the hand there is a cephalad longitudinal movement of the radius in relation to the ulna. Similarly, during ulnar deviation of the wrist there is a caudad longitudinal movement of the radius in relation to the ulna.

WRIST JOINT

It is advisable when learning movements and techniques to practise using an articulated set of bones.

The passive movements of the wrist (that is, the radiocarpal joint) are flexion, extension, radial and ulnar deviation, supination and pronation, medial and lateral transverse movements, postero-anterior and anteroposterior movements, distraction and compression. Treatment of any individual joint is often possible by general movements which affect them all. However, during examination and treatment it is necessary to differentiate between the joints.

EXAMINATION

The wrist joint is not as simple to examine accurately as one may at first feel and this is why it is useful when practising to have an articulated hand alongside. The wrist joint's movements are intimately related to the inferior radio-ulnar joint and the intercarpal joints; Table 7.6 (page 159) outlines the wrist joint and Table 7.10 (page 183) outlines examination for all the associated joints.

QUICK TESTS

To discern the extent and strength which will be required of examination movements three passive movements should be carried out. These movements are performed by moving the radiocarpal joint slowly to the limit of each range and then gently applying overpressure. If the range is good and pain is minimal the strength of the overpressure should be increased. If the movement is still comparatively pain free then a full-range amplitude movement (grade III+) should be carried out.

The method described above should be applied to the four movements in turn: first to flexion and extension as depicted in *Figures 7.25* and *7.26* (page 160); second to radial and ulnar deviation as shown in *Figure 7.29* (page 163); and third to supination and pronation as shown in *Figures 7.30* and *7.31* (pages 164 and 165). Supination and pronation occurring at the wrist joint are not described in the text but they are movements which are very important to the normal function of the wrist. The technique used to differentiate between pain arising from the inferior radio-ulnar joint and that from the wrist joint will be described in the 'Method' for each movement.

SPECIAL TESTS

In the section 'Accessory movements — As applicable' of Table 7.6 reference is made to 'differentiating' for flexion, extension, supination and pronation. In relation to flexion and extension it is sometimes necessary to know whether pain felt on flexion or extension of the hand is coming from the radiocarpal joint or the intercarpal joints. It is possible to differentiate between the two. In the description of radiocarpal flexion (page 161) emphasis is placed on grasping the proximal row of the patient's carpus. Pain felt with localized movement of the radiocarpal joint is then compared with the pain felt when the whole hand is flexed.

When pain is felt on passively stretching supination or pronation, it is necessary to determine whether the pain arises from supination of the wrist joint or from the inferior radio-ulnar joint. The patient's area of pain may be vague and therefore not helpful in making such differentiation. This same problem of 'differentiating' may occur if full pronation is painful.

When supination is painful, the technique used to differentiate between the inferior radio-ulnar and the wrist joint as the source of the pain is as follows. The forearm and hand are fully supinated as shown in *Figure 7.30* (page 164). Once in this position the patient is questioned in regard to the site and degree of pain. The physiotherapist releases her grip with her left hand while maintaining supination, with her right hand holding the patient's carpus. She must ensure that the patient's pain has not changed. At this stage she assesses the strength of the pressure required to maintain the supination stretch with her right hand. The next step is a very delicate manoeuvre. It is absolutely essential to maintain the same degree of pressure holding the supination with the right hand while she then grasps the distal ends of the radius and ulna in her left hand. She then, very minimally, pronates the inferior radio-ulnar joint with her left hand. At the same instant she asks the patient whether the degree of pain has increased or decreased.

If the pain has increased then the source of the pain lies in the radiocarpal joint.
If the pain has decreased then the fault lies within the inferior radio-ulnar joint.

If the patient has pain with both supination and pronation then exactly the same test as described above can be applied with the forearm in full pronation.

It is interesting to note that Mennell[1] shows radiographs of wrist flexion and extension which he states verify the fact that extension occurs mainly at the mid-carpal joint whereas flexion occurs at the radiocarpal joint. *Gray's Anatomy* (35th edition) states the opposite: 'When the wrist is flexed, both the radiocarpal and the midcarpal joints are implicated but the range of movement is greater at the latter. In extension the reverse is the case and most of the movement takes place at the radiocarpal joint.'[2] This statement is also substantiated by radiological evidence.

[1] Mennell, John M. (1964). *Joint Pain,* pp. 46–48. London; Churchill
[2] *Gray's Anatomy* (1973). 35th edition, p. 438. Edinburgh; Churchill Livingstone

Table 7.6
Wrist Joint: Objective Examination

[The routine examination of this joint must include inferior R/U joint and inter-carpal joints]

Observation

Active movements
 Active quick tests
 Routinely
  F, E, Ab, Ad, Sup, Pron
  Note range, pain, repeated and rapid
  Clenching fist

Static tests

Other structures in 'plan'
 As applicable
  Full active resisted movement through range for 'sheaths'

Passive movements
Physiological movements
 Routinely
  F, E, radial and ulnar deviation, Sup and Pron, ←→ceph and caud
  Note range, pain, resistance, spasm and behaviour

Accessory movements
 Routinely ↓ , ↑ , —→ , ←—

 As applicable
  1. F and E differentiating
  2. Sup and Pron differentiating
  3. Meniscus
  4. Pisiform
  5. Wrist ↑ , ↓ , —→, ←— in supination, neutral and pronation

Palpation
 Include tendon sheaths

Check case records etc.

HIGHLIGHT MAIN FINDINGS WITH ASTERISKS

After treatment

TECHNIQUES

Flexion (General)**

Starting position

The physiotherapist stands by the patient's right side beyond his flexed elbow and grasps around the medial border of his right hand with her right hand, placing her thumb against the dorsum of his metacarpals and her fingers in his palm. With her left hand immediately proximal to his carpus, she stabilizes his forearm midway between supination and pronation (*Figure 7.25*).

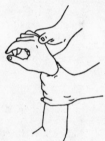

Figure 7.25.—Wrist joint; flexion (general)

Method

Starting from a position midway between flexion and extension she flexes his wrist to the limit of the range with her right thumb and returns it to the starting position with her fingers. It is her index finger, positioned near his metacarpophalangeal joints, which controls most of the returning movement.

Extension (General)**

The starting position is identical with that described above for flexion and the method involves extending the patient's wrist from the mid position to the fully extended position with her fingers, and returning it to the starting position with her thumb (*Figure 7.26*).

Figure 7.26. — Wrist joint; extension (general)

Radiocarpal flexion***

To exclude intercarpal and carpometacarpal movement from wrist flexion and extension the technique involves holding the carpus and not the metacarpals. Grades II and III are the movements most commonly employed.

Starting position

The physiotherapist stands by the patient's right hip facing his right shoulder and holds his supinated and extended arm at the wrist with both hands. His forearm is supinated for convenience but should not be held at the limit of the range. She holds with both thumbs pointing proximally on the anterior surface of the carpus and her fingers across the back of the carpus with the flexed index fingers forming the main point of contact against the proximal row of the carpus posteriorly. The index fingers and thumbs grasp the scaphoid and lunate mainly but also the triquetrum immediately opposite each other. When the grip is held firmly, the thumb contact is through the tip of the terminal phalanx rather than the base (*Figure 7.27*).

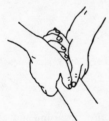

Figure 7.27. – Wrist joint; radiocarpal flexion

The grasp of the proximal row of the carpus must be very precise. When using this method of producing localized flexion (and it applies equally to radiocarpal extension, page 162) the source of joint pain can be determined very accurately if the physiotherapist grasps only the scaphoid or only the lunate, so that the fulcrum of the flexion (or extension) is even more localized. The precision of this test can be carried even further by grasping only the scaphoid while producing the flexion (or extension) and varying the point of contact between the scaphoid and the radius with the wrist in varying degrees of ulnar deviation or radial deviation. The same principle applies if the physiotherapist holds only the lunate between her fingers and thumbs.

Method

From a position midway between flexion and extension, the patient's wrist is moved downward towards the floor while the carpus, held firmly between the physiotherapist's index fingers and thumbs, is flexed on the radius and ulna. While performing this movement the carpus must be held firmly.

Radiocarpal extension***

This movement is identical with that described for radiocarpal flexion except that the patient's forearm is pronated and the physiotherapist's thumbs hold the posterior surface of the proximal row of the carpal bones while her fingers hold the proximal row of the carpal bones anteriorly. The extension movement is produced through a very firm localized grasp with fingers and thumbs while lowering the wrist towards the floor as the wrist is extended. The oscillation is produced by returning the patient's arm to the starting position while at the same time returning the extended radiocarpal joint to the mid position (*Figure 7.28*).

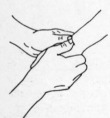

Figure 7.28. – Wrist joint; radiocarpal extension

As described in detail for radiocarpal flexion, the extension movement can be similarly localized more precisely by performing the extension grasping only the scaphoid or the lunate. Similarly the movement can be further refined by holding the wrist in varying degrees of radial and ulnar deviation.

Ulnar deviation**

Starting position

The physiotherapist stands by the patient's right shoulder, facing his feet. With her left hand she grasps his forearm distally so that her

index finger stabilizes around the styloid process of the ulna. She
flexes his elbow to 90 degrees and positions his forearm midway
between supination and pronation. With her right hand she grasps the
posterior surface of the metacarpals with her fingers reaching around
the ulnar border of his hand and her thumb through the interosseous
space (*Figure 7.29*).

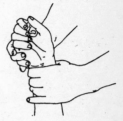

Figure 7.29. – Wrist joint; ulnar deviation

Method

The oscillatory treatment movement, performed in any part of the
range, is produced by supination of the physiotherapist's right forearm,
returning it to the starting position by a pronation movement.

Radial deviation**

The starting position is identical with that described for ulnar deviation
with the exception that now her left thumb holds around the styloid
process of the radius. The only difference in the method is that the
movement is one of radial deviation produced by pronation of the
physiotherapist's right forearm.

Radiocarpal supination***

Starting position

The physiotherapist stands by the patient's flexed and supinated right
forearm. She holds his forearm adjacent to the wrist with her left hand
so that her thumb hooks around the lateral border of the distal end of
the radius to reach the posterior surface of the radius. Her index
finger makes firm contact against the anterior surface of the distal end
of the ulna. With her right hand she holds across the posterior surface
of the proximal row of his carpus so that her thumb hooks around the

scaphoid to hold it firmly anteriorly while her index finger lies across the proximal row of the carpal bones posteriorly making the firmest contact against the triquetrum (*Figure 7.30*).

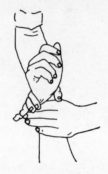

Figure 7.30. – Wrist joint; radio-carpal supination

Method

Further supination of the radio-ulnar joint is prevented by the physio-therapist's left hand while the added supination of the radiocarpal joint is produced by her right arm acting through her wrist and hand. The tip of her right thumb and the distal end of the proximal phalanx of her index finger are the points through which all of the pressure is transmitted to the carpus while her left thumb and index finger provide counterpressure.

Although radiocarpal supination has been described with the forearm supinated, it can be performed with the forearm anywhere between full supination and full pronation.

Radiocarpal pronation*

Starting position

The physiotherapist stands by the patient's right hip, facing his shoulder. With his elbow flexed to a right angle she holds the distal end of his forearm in her right hand with her thumb hooked posteriorly around his ulna and the base of her index finger against the anterior surface of the radius. With her left hand she grasps around the carpus, her thumb holding around the triquetral bone anteriorly and her index finger pressed firmly against the posterior surface of the scaphoid (*Figure 7.31*).

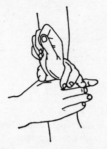

Figure 7.31. – Wrist joint; radio-carpal pronation

Method

The movement is produced by the physiotherapist's left hand against the carpus while her right hand stabilizes the patient's forearm by applying an equal and opposite counterpressure.

Postero-anterior movement***

Postero-anterior movement of the carpus on the radius is mainly used in the treatment of stiff joints rather than extremely painful joints. Therefore, grades III and IV are the movements most commonly used.

Starting position

The physiotherapist stands by the patient's right hip, facing his head, and holds his forearm midway between supination and pronation. She holds the posterior surface of his hand in her left hand and the anterior surface of his distal forearm in her right hand which is fully supinated and extended at the wrist and pointing proximally. The heel of her left hand should lie over the carpus, her fingers grasping around his thumb and her thumb grasping around the ulnar border of his hand. The heel of her right hand is placed level with the distal end of his radius and ulna while her fingers grasp around his forearm. She should crouch over his arm to direct her forearms opposite each other (*Figure 7.32*).

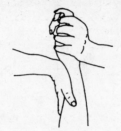

Figure 7.32. — Wrist joint; postero-anterior movement

Method

If a grade III movement is employed the oscillation starts from the neutral position and is taken to the limit of the range by an equal and opposite movement of the forearm. It is important to keep the patient's hand straight to prevent any flexion or extension of his wrist. Grade IV movements are performed through a much smaller amplitude at the limit of the range.

Anteroposterior movement***

Starting position

The physiotherapist stands between the patient's right side and his elbow and faces away from him. His elbow is flexed and supported midway between supination and pronation. She grasps his palm from

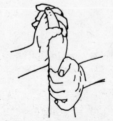

Figure 7.33. — Wrist joint; antero-posterior movement

in front with her right hand, her thumb holding around the ulnar border of his hand and her fingers around the radial border. His thumb lies between her ring and middle fingers. The heel of her hand forms the main point of contact against his carpus anteriorly. She places the base of her left thumb opposite the distal border of the radius posteriorly and grasps around his radius with her fingers (*Figure 7.33*). This technique can also be performed using the edge of the couch as a fulcrum.

Method

The method for this technique resembles that described above for postero-anterior movement.

Lateral transverse movement***

Starting position

The patient lies supine with his arm abducted. His wrist lies at the edge of the couch with his hand beyond it and his thumb pointing towards the floor. With her left hand the physiotherapist holds firmly around the distal end of his radius and ulna, immediately around the styloid processes. Her knuckles, between the patient's distal forearm and the surface of the couch, stabilize his wrist but it may be necessary for her to rest her forearm across his forearm or elbow to stabilize the arm.

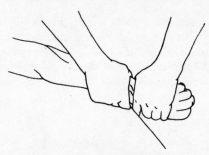

*Figure 7.34. – Wrist joint; lateral trans-
verse movement*

With her right hand she grasps around the posterior surface of his hand so that her thumb and index finger grasp the carpus immediately adjacent to the proximal end of the first metacarpal and the pisiform (*Figure 7.34*).

Method

Movement of the patient's hand towards the floor is produced through the physiotherapist's left arm and shoulder. Proper movement can only be gained if the physiotherapist's left hand moves as a single unit with the patient's hand.

The movement can be performed as an oscillatory grade IV to IV+ or as a large amplitude grade III.

Four variations can be made with the technique. These changes would be indicated when any one of them more exactly reproduced the patient's symptoms. The variations are as follows:

1. The patient's hand can be positioned in any degree of ulnar or radial deviation and held in this position while the transverse movement is produced.
2. The direction of the radial transverse movement can be inclined posteriorly or anteriorly, where, although the available range is smaller it may more accurately produce the comparable pain.
3. The wrist may be positioned in any degree of supination or pronation prior to applying the transverse movement.
4. The transverse movement may be performed with a degree of compression of the intercarpal and radiocarpal joint surfaces or the joint surfaces may be distracted during transverse movement.

Medial transverse movement***

Starting position

The patient lies supine and abducts his arm so that his wrist is at the edge of the table. The physiotherapist grasps above and below the wrist as in the previous technique but this time the patient's thumb is pointing towards the ceiling (*Figure 7.35*) instead of towards the floor.

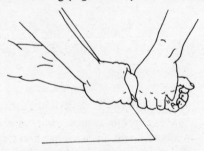

Figure 7.35. – Wrist joint; medial trans-verse movement

Method

The technique is identical with that described for the previous movement and the emphasis is on the fact that the patient's hand and the
physiotherapist's hand move as a single unit.

The variations listed above in numbers 1–4 apply in exactly the
same manner in this technique.

INTERCARPAL MOVEMENT

EXAMINATION

The bones, joints and movements of the carpus are complex (*Figure
7.36*) yet it is surprising how, with skill, it is possible to assess the
range of movement and the behaviour of pain between each of the

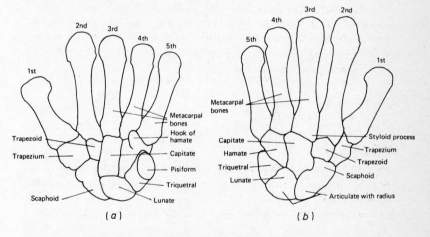

*Figure 7.36. (a) The carpal and metacarpal bones of the left hand. Palmar aspect.
(b) The carpal and metacarpal bones of the left hand. Dorsal aspect. (Reproduced
by courtesy of* Gray's Anatomy *(1973), pp. 336, 337. 35th Edition. Edinburgh;
Churchill Livingstone)*

bones. Because of this, if the treatment technique is localized to the
particularly restricted and painful movement, the result will be
achieved much more quickly than if general hand and wrist movements
are used. As was shown and explained in Chapter 2 (*Figures 2.1–2.6*,
pages 22–24), the tests are intricate and require care and skill.

QUICK TESTS

There are no specific quick tests for the carpus other than to ask the patient to flick his hand into full flexion, full extension, full radial and ulnar deviation, and full supination and pronation. It is also useful to ask him to make a fist while the physiotherapist assesses movement and strength.

SPECIAL TESTS

The first of the special tests is to hold one carpal bone between the fingers and thumb of one hand while the other hand holds and moves the adjacent carpal bone to assess whether the ranges of anteroposterior and postero-anterior movement are full and painless.

The second of the special tests consists of the postero-anteriorly directed pressures (which may be varied with a caudad, cephalad, medial and lateral inclination) on each of the two bones and then the joint space as described in Chapter 2 on Examination (pages 22–24).

Table 7.7 lists the examination by passive movements.

When considering the carpus it must not be forgotten that the pisiform, which articulates with the triquetrum and has the ulnar nerve immediately adjacent to its radial surface, is also capable of movements which should be tested.

TECHNIQUES

Intercarpal horizontal extension**

Starting position

The physiotherapist stands by the patient's right side, beyond his flexed and supinated forearm, facing his head. She holds his right hand from the back with the tips of the pads of her thumbs against the centre of the carpus posteriorly and her index and middle fingers around the pisiform medially and the carpometacarpal joint of the thumb laterally (*Figure 7.37*).

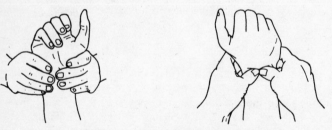

Figure 7.37. – Intercarpal horizontal extension

Table 7.7
Intercarpal Joints: Objective Examination

[The routine examination of these joints must also include examination of the wrist joint and carpometacarpal (C/MC) joints]

Observation

Active movements
    Active quick tests as described for wrist joint

Static tests

Other structures in 'plan'
    Add full active resisted movement through range for 'sheaths'

Passive movements
Physiological movements
    Routinely
    1. Wrist F, E, Ab, Ad
    2. Differentiating F and E
    3. Individual C/MC F and E
    Note range, pain, resistance, spasm and behaviour

Accessory movements
    Routinely
    1. ↓ and ↕ (varying angles), ↕ (i.e. gliding of each carpal bone on adjacent carpal bone) with and without compression
    2. HF and HE of carpus
    3. Pisiform
    4. C/MC joints
        (a) ↓ and ↕ (varying angles), ↕
        (b) →• , •← of metacarpals on carpus, with and without abduction and adduction
        (c) ↺ and ↻ metacarpals
    Note range, pain, resistance, spasm and behaviour

Palpation
    Include tendon sheaths

Check case records etc.

HIGHLIGHT MAIN FINDINGS WITH ASTERISKS

After treatment

Method

The oscillatory movement is produced by thumb pressure against the centre of the carpus posteriorly and pulling against the medial and lateral margins of the carpus with her fingers. This action is produced by extension of the physiotherapist's wrists which is facilitated by pushing the patient's hand away from her.

Variations

The movement as described so far is a general one involving the full length and breadth of the carpus. For examination purposes it may be found that the general horizontal extension is pain free. When this is so, the tips of the thumbs should localize the fulcrum of the movement by limiting their point of contact to each carpal bone in both the proximal and distal rows.

With experience and practice, it is possible to determine that an individual carpal bone cannot be moved anteriorly as far as its normal range or that it may be hypermobile. By altering the fulcrum of the horizontal extension to each of the bones, one will, when pushed anteriorly, reproduce the patient's pain. It may well be that this joint sign is the main 'comparable' sign and therefore may be the technique used in treatment. It should also be pointed out that this localization of the movement will divulge whether it is a hypermobile or a hypomobile joint causing the pain.

The postero-anteriorly directed pressures should be inclined medially, laterally, cephalad, caudad and also diagonally between these limits. These variations can be in any direction. They have been described in Chapter 2 (pages 22–24).

Intercarpal horizontal flexion**

The intercarpal horizontal flexion movement is not as useful as extension because the movement is less frequently restricted or painful.

Starting position

The physiotherapist stands by the patient's right elbow, facing across his body, and supports his supinated and flexed forearm by grasping the back of his hand in her right hand with her fingers pointing distally.

The main contact with her right hand is at the medial and lateral margins of the carpus. She places her left thumb tip against the palmar surface of the carpus to apply a direct anteroposterior pressure. This fulcrum provided by her left thumb would first be used on the proximal row and then the distal row of the carpus. She then directs both forearms opposite each other (*Figure 7.38*).

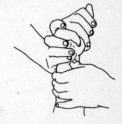

Figure 7.38. – Intercarpal horizontal flexion

Method

The oscillation is produced by opposite pressure through the forearms. The right hand produces a cupping action of the patient's hand around the pivot formed by the physiotherapist's left thumb.

Variations

The same variations in regard to the point of contact as described for intercarpal horizontal extension (page 172) should be used. This also applies to the direction of the thumb pressure, referred to as postero-anterior, which should also be varied in inclination as described on page 23.

Postero-anterior intercarpal movement***

Localized intercarpal movements are extremely effective as treatment techniques when the movement is painful.

Starting position

The patient lies with his pronated hand resting on the couch. The physiotherapist stands by his right side, beyond his hand, and places her thumb tips, adjacent to each other, on the appropriate carpal bone or intercarpal joint. She spreads her fingers over the adjacent area of the hand for stability (*Figure 7.39*). She then directs her arms and thumbs either immediately postero-anteriorly or combined with any of the inclinations described in detail on page 23.

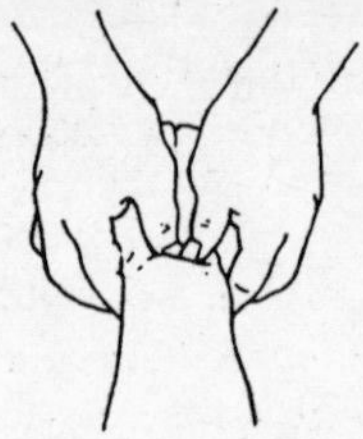

Figure 7.39. – *Postero-anterior intercarpal movement*

Method

Postero-anterior mobilizing is produced by pressure from the physiotherapist's arms transmitted through the spring-like action of the thumbs against the carpal bone or intercarpal joint.

Anteroposterior intercarpal movement*

Anteroposterior movement is similarly produced but the thumb contact is against the palmar surface of the patient's supinated hand although the individual carpal bones are much harder to find anteriorly (*Figure 7.40*).

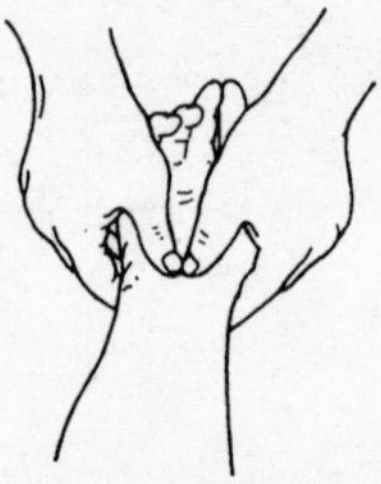

Figure 7.40. – *Anteroposterior intercarpal movement*

Both anteroposterior and postero-anterior pressures can be used in conjunction with wrist flexion or extension emphasizing the movement of a particular intercarpal joint.

Longitudinal movement caudad*

The distraction technique has been described (*see* page 146, *Figure 7.21*) but when it is used to treat the carpus the physiotherapist must ensure that her grasp surrounds the metacarpals and not the carpus. Also, the movement can be emphasized more to the medial, central or lateral, mid-carpal joints by using the index finger to distract the lateral mid-carpal joint and so on.

Longitudinal movement cephalad*

The compression technique has been described (*see* page 147, *Figure 7.22*), but with the patient's wrist in extension. To meet the present aim the physiotherapist should grasp more distally and hold firmly around the medial four metacarpals. The compression is then transferred through his intercarpal joints. Though the technique is depicted in a neutral wrist position (*Figure 7.41*) the patient's wrist may be positioned anywhere between flexion and extension, radial and ulnar deviation. Also, as has been described above, each of the patient's fingers may be used so as to localize the compression to different intercarpal joints.

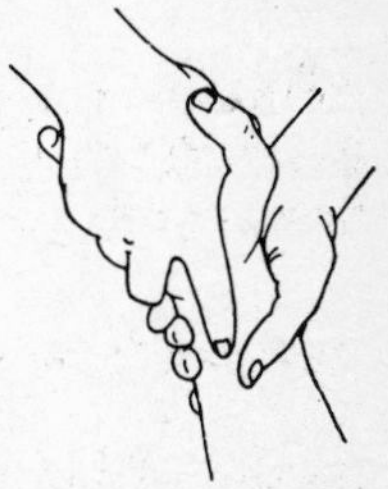

Figure 7.41. – Intercarpal longitudinal movement

This technique is not used alone but has considerable application in treatment when used in conjunction with other intercarpal movements. For example, if pain arises from the joint between the capitate and lunate, the only 'comparable sign' may be a rocking anteroposterior to postero-anterior movement directed against the joint line while compression is added in a cephalad direction through the third metacarpal. This example is only one of innumerable variations where the direction of pressure through different angles against different points on the carpus may be used as test movements and treatment movements.

Pisiform movement

It is not often that movement between the pisiform and the triquetral bone is limited, thickened or inflamed, resulting in symptoms. However, there are times when movement of the pisiform is restricted and does irritate the ulnar nerve which is adjacent to its lateral surface. The movement can be mobilized just as any moving part can be.

Starting position

With the patient lying supine, his arm outstretched and the back of his hand resting on the treatment couch, the physiotherapist maintains stability of the hand and forearm while directing pressure against the different surfaces of the pisiform to make it move on the triquetral bone. To make the mobilizing techniques comfortable she should use as much of the pad of her thumb as possible, though not at the expense of localizing the contact point, so that the direction of movement can be finely varied from one direction to another.

Method

Movement of the pisiform is produced through the thumb by pressure from the physiotherapist's arm. The movement is an oscillatory one and in treatment usually needs to be a grade IV type movement (*Figure 7.42*).

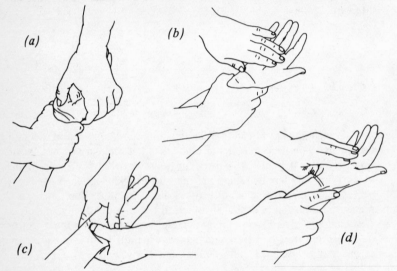

Figure 7.42. – Pisiform movement (a) cephalad; (b) caudad; (c) medially; (d) laterally

Variations

It is quite usual to vary the direction of the pressure against the pisiform, moving it in any direction which may stretch into the limitation of movement or reproduce the patient's symptoms. Previously, variations have been described for the different directions of movement. However, in relation to the pisiform it is necessary to remember that the different directions of movement can also be combined with compression of the pisiform against the triquetral bone. Coincidentally, distraction of the pisiform can be produced by gripping all sides of the pisiform and lifting it from the triquetrum by squeezing all fingers towards the central point inside the joint.

TREATMENT

It is common, with falls that result in fractures of the radius and ulna, for the hand also to be sprained or strained. During examination, therefore, movements of the intercarpal joints should be included. Pain found on movement of any intercarpal joint or joints should be part of follow-up treatment when the arm is taken out of plaster. General movements of the wrist and hand should be used both as grade IV— and as grade II, II+ or III. Where abnormal or painful movement can be localized to one joint the technique used should be localized to that joint rather than performed as a general movement of all carpal bones.

Carpal tunnel syndrome

This syndrome can sometimes be relieved by direct anteroposterior pressure, where the pressure reproduces the patient's symptoms. Also, the technique (shown on page 170, *Figure 7.37*) can be used to stretch the

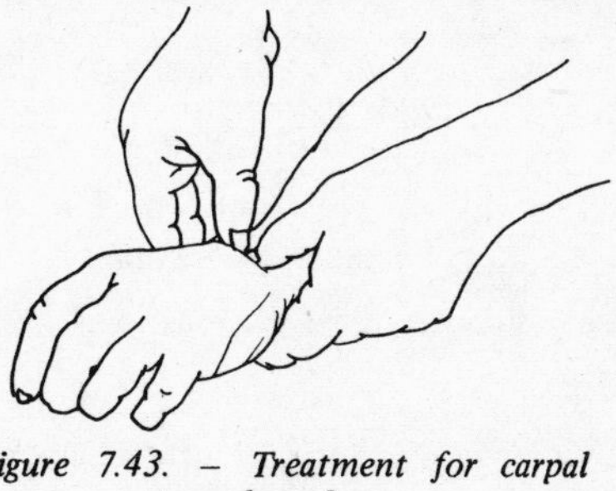

Figure 7.43. — Treatment for carpal tunnel syndrome

flexor retinaculum. While the fingers of each hand separate the pisiform and the hook of the hamate away from the trapezium and scaphoid, the thumb tips on the posterior surface of the carpus form a fulcrum for the movement. If the patient's symptoms can be reproduced by localizing the pressure to one bone on the posterior surfaces of the carpus, then this bone should be used as the fulcrum point for treatment technique. To determine whether this reproduction of symptoms is possible, the tips of the thumbs should be used as the fulcrum for the horizontal extension movement on the capitate and the lunate first. Pressure should then be applied through the trapezoid, the hamate, the triquetrum and the scaphoid. The pressure can be inclined in any direction in an effort to find the exact movement for the treatment (*Figure 7.43*).

CARPOMETACARPAL JOINTS

The description is here confined to the fingers; the thumb is described separately with the remainder of its movements (*see* pages 197–202). Table 7.8 provides the examination movements.

Table 7.8
Carpometacarpal Joints: Objective Examination

[The routine examination of these joints must include examination of intercarpal joints, and proximal and distal intermetacarpal joints and spaces]

Observation

Active movements
> Active quick tests
> as described for wrist joint

Static tests

Other joints in 'plan'

Passive movements
Physiological movements
> Routinely
>> Individual C/MC F and E
>> HF and HE of carpus
>> HF and HE of metacarpals } and differentiating
>> Note range, pain, resistance, spasm and behaviour

Accessory movements
> Routinely
>> 1. ↕ and ↕ (varying angles), ↕ of metacarpals on carpus
>> 2. ⟶ and ⟵
>> 3. Abduction and adduction
>> 4. Combining (2) with (3)
>> 5. ↺ and ↻ of metacarpals
>> 6. Add compression to 1–5 as necessary
>> Note range, resistance, pain, spasm and behaviour

Palpation
> Include tendon sheaths

Check case records etc.

HIGHLIGHT MAIN FINDINGS WITH ASTERISKS

After treatment

Extension***

Starting position

The supine position for the patient is still the position of choice because better relaxation is possible than if he sits. If the lateral carpometacarpal joints are to be mobilized, the physiotherapist stands by his slightly flexed right forearm facing across his body. She holds his partially pronated hand in her hands, grasping from the medial side, the relevant carpal bone in her left hand and the relevant metacarpal in her right. Her right hand grasps through the first interosseous space and the tip of her right thumb is placed against the base of the metacarpal posteriorly (*Figure 7.44a*).

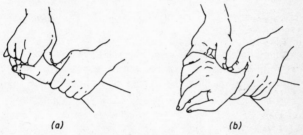

(a)   (b)

Figure 7.44. – Carpometacarpal extension (a) of index finger;
(b) of little finger

When mobilizing the carpometacarpal joint of the little finger the physiotherapist maintains the same grip with her left hand except that she places the pad of her thumb over the patient's hamate. With her right hand she holds around the ulnar border of the patient's right hand to grasp the fifth metacarpal, her flexed index finger supporting it distally and anteriorly and her thumb contacting the base posteriorly (*Figure 7.44b*).

Method

Grades III and IV are the movements most commonly used with this technique. The movement is produced by the physiotherapist moving the patient's hand away from her and applying pressure through her thumbs while applying a pulling counterpressure with her fingers to assist the extension. This movement can be performed either in large amplitude (grade III) or small amplitude oscillations (grade IV).

Flexion***

Starting position

The physiotherapist stands by the patient's upper arm, facing his feet, and holds his supinated hand in her hands. She holds around the medial border of his wrist with her left hand, placing the tip of her thumb in his palm over the appropriate carpal bone. If the carpometacarpal joint of the index finger is to be mobilized she holds the second metacarpal

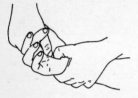

Figure 7.45. – *Carpometacarpal flexion*

through the first interosseous space in her right hand. She places the tip of her thumb against the base of the metacarpal anteriorly and her flexed index finger against the posterior surface of the metacarpal distally (*Figure 7.45*).

Method

The physiotherapist produces the movement by pushing the patient's hand away from her at the same time as adducting her glenohumeral joints and extending her elbows to transmit pressure through her thumbs to his palm.

The movement of flexion can be produced by the movement of both hands as described above, or it may be produced by stabilizing the carpus with the left hand and flexing the metacarpal with the right hand.

Accessory movements***

The grip for each carpometacarpal joint has been described and related to the movements of flexion and extension.

Other movements can be produced at this joint by inclining the direction of pressure techniques against the face of the metacarpal bone. The direction of this pressure may be inclined medially or laterally.

If the tip of the right thumb can be wedged between adjacent metacarpal bones, a transverse pressure can be exerted on the metacarpal bone through the tip of the thumb. Although very little movement can be felt, comparison with the other hand makes it possible to assess range. Also, it may reproduce the patient's symptoms and this may guide the physiotherapist to use this direction of movement as the treatment movement.

Rotation of the carpometacarpal joint can be obtained by flexing to 90 degrees the relevant metacarpophalangeal joint and then rotating the metacarpal by swinging the flexed finger medially and laterally.

The base of the metacarpal can also be made to move anteroposteriorly and postero-anteriorly in relation to the adjacent metacarpal and the carpal bone with which it articulates.

The carpometacarpal joint may also be distracted or compressed and while in this position the other movements described above may be incorporated. When the carpometacarpal joint causes pain the test movements performed while the joint is compressed are most likely to reproduce a 'comparable sign'.

The transverse movement, the rotary movements and the antero-posterior and postero-anterior movements can also be produced in conjunction with different positions of flexion, extension, radial and ulnar deviation.

TREATMENT

The techniques used in the treatment of the carpometacarpal joints are similar to those described for the intercarpal joints. That is, by varying the angles of movements of the carpometacarpal joints, if one is found to be more restricted than the comparable joint of the other hand and this restricted movement reproduces the patient's symptoms then grade IV type movements should be used to increase the range. Any treatment soreness produced by this technique would be relieved by continuing the same movement but producing a grade III— type technique.

INTERMETACARPAL MOVEMENT

The main movements between the metacarpals involve cupping and flattening of the palm (which are perhaps better thought of as horizontal flexion and horizontal extension, respectively), and the parallel antero-posterior and postero-anterior movements of one metacarpal relative to its neighbouring metacarpal. Though the movements are similar they are not identical.

EXAMINATION

The localized techniques described are the only special tests for this area. The examination is given in Table 7.9.

Table 7.10 is a guide to a composite examination of the joints from the inferior radio-ulnar joint to the carpometacarpal joints. The differentiating of supination and pronation refers to holding the patient's hand and forearm fully supinated to reproduce his pain. While maintaining this position and degree of pain, the physiotherapist pronates

Table 7.9
Intermetacarpal Movement: Objective Examination

Observation

Active movements
   Active quick tests, localized HF, and HE

Other structures in 'plan'
   Full active resisted movement through range for 'sheaths'

Static tests (not applicable)

Passive movements
Physiological movements
   Routinely
      HF and HE of metacarpals
      Note range, pain, resistance, spasm and behaviour
Accessory movements
   Routinely
      ↓ and ↑ of each metacarpal in relation to its neighbour (on bases and heads)
      Note range, resistance, pain, spasm and behaviour
   As applicable
      1. Individual HF or HE (bases and heads)
      2. Individual ↓ or ↑

Palpation
   Include tendon sheaths

Check case records etc.

HIGHLIGHT MAIN FINDINGS WITH ASTERISKS

After treatment

Table 7.10
Composite Wrist/Hand: Objective Examination

Observation

Active quick tests
    Clench fist and test grip
    F, E, Ab and Ad of wrist
    Sup and Pron

Static tests

Other joints in 'plan'

Passive tests
    Routinely
      Whole hand
      1. F and E
      2. Radial and ulnar deviation
      3. Supination and pronation
      4. ←•→ ceph and caud
      5. HF and HE
      6. Pisiform
      7. ↕ , ↑ , →•→ , ←•→ , in different positions of wrist Sup and Pron,
         F and E
    Differentiating as required
      1. F and E
        (*a*) radiocarpal
        (*b*) midcarpal
        (*c*) carpometacarpal
      2. Radial and ulnar deviation
        (*a*) radiocarpal
        (*b*) midcarpal
        (*c*) carpometacarpal
      3. Supination and pronation
        (*a*) radiocarpal
        (*b*) inferior R/U joint
      4. ←•→ caud and ceph
        (*a*) radiocarpal
        (*b*) intercarpal
        (*c*) carpometacarpal
      5. HF and HE
        (*a*) intercarpal
        (*b*) carpometacarpal
        (*c*) intermetacarpal
    Other test movements

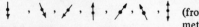 (from inferior R/U to heads of metacarpals)

    Add compression as required

Palpation

Check case records etc.

HIGHLIGHT MAIN FINDINGS WITH ASTERISKS

After treatment

the inferior radio-ulnar joint. If the patient's pain decreases, the source of the pain is the inferior radio-ulnar joint. If the pain increases, the supinated wrist is the source.

General horizontal flexion*

Starting position

When the horizontal flexion movement is performed as a general movement for the whole row of metacarpals the physiotherapist places the pad of her left thumb pointing distally in his palm over the distal end of the third metacarpal while cupping her right hand across the dorsum of all the metacarpals distally. Her right thumb presses against the posterior surface of the second metacarpal and her fingers, particularly her index fingers, press against the posterior surface of the fifth metacarpal (*Figure 7.46*).

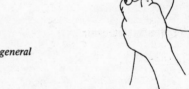

Figure 7.46. – Intermetacarpal general horizontal flexion

Method

Small or large amplitude oscillations are produced by moving the hands in opposite directions.

The same movement can be localized to two adjacent metacarpals but the technique differs slightly.

Localized horizontal flexion**

Starting position

The physiotherapist stands facing the back of the patient's supinated and flexed forearm and grasps his hand with her two hands. She does this by holding the medial metacarpal posteriorly with her right thumb posteriorly, and anteriorly with the tips of her index and middle fingers. With her left hand she holds the adjacent metacarpal between the pads of her index and middle fingers anteriorly and the pad of her thumb posteriorly (*Figure 7.47*).

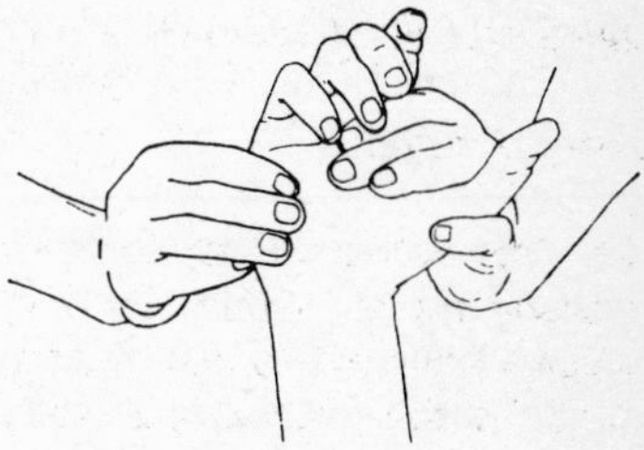

Figure 7.47. – Intermetacarpal localized horizontal flexion

Method

While her left hand stabilizes one metacarpal she moves the other with her right hand in a circular direction around it. When the second metacarpal is mobilized on the third, the physiotherapist's left hand performs the movement, whereas when the fourth and fifth metacarpals are mobilized her left hand holds the fourth metacarpal while her right hand moves the fifth metacarpal around the fourth. It really does not matter whether it is done as described or in reverse.

General horizontal extension*

Starting position

The physiotherapist stands beyond the patient's flexed and supinated forearm facing the back of his hand which she holds in her two hands. She places the pads of her thumbs against the distal end of the posterior surface of the third metacarpal. With her fingers she holds around the medial and lateral margins of his hand to reach the anterior surface of the second and fifth metacarpals distally (*Figure 7.48*).

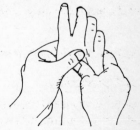

Figure 7.48. – Intermetacarpal general horizontal extension

Method

The extension movement is performed by a pulling action with the fingers of both hands pivoting the patient's metacarpals around the thumbs on the third metacarpal while at the same time pushing his hand away. This can be done as a large amplitude grade III movement or as a small movement at the limit of the range (grade IV).

Localized horizontal extension**

This movement can also be localized to two adjacent metacarpals and is performed with the same grasp as that described for localized metacarpal horizontal flexion (*Figure 7.47*), except that the action is one of pivoting towards extension around the stabilized adjacent metacarpal (*Figure 7.49*).

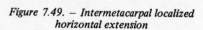

*Figure 7.49. – Intermetacarpal localized
horizontal extension*

Postero-anterior and anteroposterior movement***

The starting position is the same as that described for localized intermetacarpal horizontal flexion and extension (*Figures 7.47* and *7.49*) and the method is similar except that instead of one metacarpal pivoting around its neighbour they traverse parallel lines moving in opposite directions. One metacarpal moves anteroposteriorly or posteroanteriorly in relation to the neighbouring metacarpal.

Compression

Starting position

The patient's hand should be grasped in a hand-shake position, that is, right hand to right hand and left to left. The physiotherapist should grip around the heads of the metacarpals and her other hand should stabilize the head of the metacarpals in a straight line from the radial to the ulnar side.

Method

The physiotherapist alternately squeezes and relaxes her grasp of the heads of the metacarpals, assessing for pain. She then compares the findings with the other hand.

TREATMENT

Movements between the metacarpals are rarely a source of pain unless the hand has been subjected to some trauma. When pain and stiffness are present, grade IV and IV+ type movements should be used, and used quite strongly.

It is more common for pain to arise from the intermetacarpal synovial joints at their bases. When this is the case the site of pain will be over the joint and the positive comparable joint signs will be among the test movements listed in Table 7.8 (page 178).

METACARPOPHALANGEAL
AND INTERPHALANGEAL JOINTS

EXAMINATION

As the techniques used for the metacarpophalangeal and interphalangeal joints of the fingers and the thumb are identical, description of the metacarpophalangeal joint of the index finger will suffice. When passive movement is used in the treatment of stiff fingers, mobilization is given in many directions and movement in one direction may be coupled with movement in other directions. For example, while the metacarpophalangeal joint of the index finger is being flexed, antero-posterior or postero-anterior mobilizing pressures may be applied to the joint. Compression may also be added to these movements. Although each movement will be described separately it must be remembered that they can be used in combination.

The only quick tests are opening wide the hand and then forming a fist. Getting the patient to squeeze the physiotherapist's hand is also informative.

Table 7.11 lists the examination for the metacarpophalangeal and interphalangeal joints.

Table 7.11
Metacarpophalangeal and Interphalangeal Joints: Objective Examination

Observation

Active movements
    Active quick tests
    Routinely
        F, E, spreading; fist/grip
        Note range and pain, repeated and rapid

Static tests

Other structures in 'plan'
    As applicable
        Full active resisted movements through range for 'sheaths'
        Joint restriction c.f. muscle/tendon restriction

Passive movements
Physiological movement
    Routinely
        F, E, Ab, Ad
        Note range, pain, resistance, spasm and behaviour
    As applicable
        Joint restriction c.f. muscle/tendon restriction
Accessory movements
    Routinely
        1. ↔ ceph and caud, Ab, Ad, ⟶ , ↞ , ⇡ , ⇣ , ↺ , ↻
        2. The above in different positions of other physiological ranges
    As applicable
        1. Same movements under compression
        2. Ab, with ⟶ and ↞
        3. Ad with ⟶ and ↞

Palpation
    Include tendon sheaths

Check case records etc.

HIGHLIGHT MAIN FINDINGS WITH ASTERISKS

After treatment

Flexion*

Starting position

The physiotherapist holds the proximal phalanx of the patient's index finger in her right hand between her thumb and index finger, both of which are directed proximally. With her left hand she stabilizes his hand, particularly around the second metacarpal, between the finger and the thumb. The joint is then flexed to the comfortable limit of the range (*Figure 7.50*).

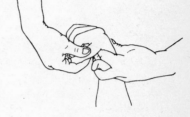

*Figure   7.50.   –   Metacarpophalangeal
               flexion*

Method

If grade IV movements are required, a small amplitude oscillation is performed with the physiotherapist's right hand while she stabilizes the metacarpal with her left. Any grade of movement can be performed with this grasp but grade I movements are rarely required.

Extension*

Starting position

This technique is the same as that described for flexion except that the metacarpophalangeal joint is comfortably extended.

Method

The oscillatory movement is produced by the combined action of extending the phalanx on the metacarpal and the metacarpal on the phalanx. Small or large oscillations can readily be produced. The movement can also be produced by stabilizing the metacarpal and moving the proximal phalanx into extension.

Abduction**

Starting position

The physiotherapist holds the posterior surface of the patient's right hand with her right hand and his index finger with her left hand. She holds the posterior surface of his hand from the radial side and places

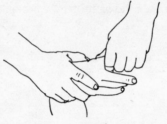

Figure   7.51.   –   Metacarpophalangeal abduction

her thumb, pointing distally, against the lateral surface of the second metacarpal distally while her fingers grasp the ulnar border of his hand. The pad of her left thumb, pointing proximally, stretches along the lateral surface of the proximal phalanx to its head (*Figure 7.51*).

Method

The oscillatory abduction produced by movement of the physio-therapist's two hands combines abduction with pushing the patient's hand away. Moving his hand away as the joint is abducted makes the mobilization easier to perform. As with other techniques small or large amplitudes in any part of the range can easily be performed.

Adduction**

Starting position

It is not as easy to hold the metacarpal during this technique as it is during abduction. The physiotherapist holds the posterior surface of the patient's hand around its radial border with her left hand, wedging as much of the tip of her thumb as she can into the second interosseous

space against the ulnar surface of the distal end of the second metacarpal. She reaches with the fingers of her left hands both around his
thumb and through the first interosseous space to stabilize his hand.
With her right hand she grips his index finger with the pad of her right
thumb, pointing proximally, against the medial surface of the proximal
phalanx (*Figure 7.52*).

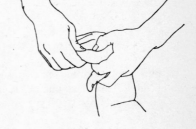

Figure 7.52. – *Metacarpophalangeal
adduction*

Method

The adduction movement is produced by the physiotherapist's arms
acting through both hands while pushing the patient's hand away from
her.

Medial rotation**

Starting position

The physiotherapist stabilizes the patient's second metacarpal with her
left hand by holding it firmly between her fingers anteriorly and her
thumb posteriorly while she holds his slightly flexed index finger in
her right hand. The metacarpophalangeal joint is flexed approximately
10 degrees and the proximal interphalangeal joint 80 degrees. She places
the tip of her right thumb against the medial aspect of the proximal
interphalangeal joint and the tips of her index and middle fingers
against the lateral surface of the middle and distal phalanges (*Figure
7.53*). The maximum range of medial rotation is obtained when the

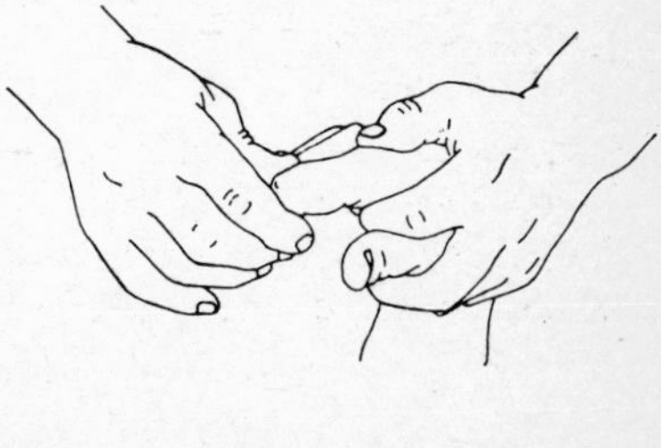

Figure 7.53. – *Metacarpophalangeal
medial rotation*

metacarpophalangeal joint is positioned in a few degrees of flexion which places it midway between its limits of flexion and extension. This is not necessarily the position in which the rotation is performed in treatment but it is the position of greatest range in a normal joint. The degree of flexion and extension in which the medial rotation is used in treatment is usually either the most restricted range of medial rotation or the most painful.

Method

The movement is produced entirely by the physiotherapist's right hand while her left hand stabilizes his hand. She pivots the distal phalanx around her thumb tip, causing the proximal phalanx to medially rotate.

Lateral rotation**

Starting position

The physiotherapist holds across the posterior surface of the patient's hand with her left hand threading her fingers around the lateral border, her index finger passing through the first interosseous space to reach the palm and her remaining fingers grasping around the thenar eminence.

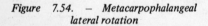

Figure   7.54.   –   Metacarpophalangeal
lateral rotation

She holds his flexed finger in her right hand with her thumb against the lateral surface of the proximal interphalangeal joint and her index finger against the medial surface of the distal interphalangeal joint (*Figure 7.54*).

Method

The physiotherapist produces the rotation by movement of her left hand and forearm while her right hand stabilizes the patient's hand.

Longitudinal movement caudad**

Starting position

The physiotherapist grasps firmly around the lateral border of the patient's right hand with her left hand and holds his index finger in her right hand. His second metacarpal, held in her left hand, is grasped between her flexed index finger threaded through the first interosseous

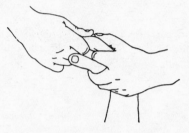

Figure   7.55.   –   Metacarpophalangeal longitudinal movement caudad

space, and her thumb so that the proximal interphalangeal joint of her index finger is against the anterior surface of the distal end of the metacarpal and her thumb is held firmly against the shaft posteriorly. With her right hand she grasps his index finger in a similar fashion, her fully flexed index finger holding the proximal phalanx anteriorly while her thumb grasps along the shaft posteriorly. His metacarpophalangeal joint is then positioned midway between its other ranges to permit maximum distraction; this usually requires a slight degree of flexion (*Figure 7.55*).

Method

While holding the metacarpophalangeal joint in a small degree of flexion the physiotherapist produces distraction by pulling her hands away from each other. The selected position of metacarpophalangeal flexion is maintained during the mobilization by firm pressure against the anterior surface of the patient's metacarpal and phalanx adjacent to the joint by her index fingers at their proximal interphalangeal joints.

Longitudinal movement cephalad*

Starting position

As described for distraction the physiotherapist holds the patient's second metacarpal firmly between her fully flexed index finger and thumb. She holds his index finger similarly except that she holds all of his index finger, slightly flexed at each interphalangeal joint, between her fingers and palm (*Figure 7.56*).

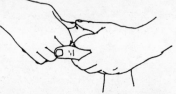

Figure 7.56. – Metacarpophalangeal longitudinal movement cephalad

Method

The movement is applied by a squeezing together of the physiotherapist's hands. During this movement it is essential to hold the metacarpal and the index finger firmly.

When the joint is the source of pain and, on examination, both active and passive physiological movements are painless, the passive movements should be repeated while the joint is compressed. One or more of these movements are commonly found to be painful. The painful movement can then be used in treatment, by making the use of the compression as described above.

Postero-anterior movement***

Starting position

The patient's second metacarpal is held firmly in the physiotherapist's left hand with her fully flexed index finger anteriorly and her thumb posteriorly. Her thumb contacts the posterior surface proximal to the joint while the proximal interphalangeal joint of her index finger contacts the anterior surface. This positioning is necessary to counter the postero-anterior pressure against the head of the phalanx. She grasps the proximal phalanx of his index finger in her right hand with her fingers hooking around the anterior surface and the tip of her thumb against the head of the proximal phalanx posteriorly (*Figure 7.57*).

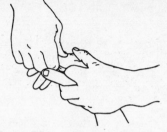

Figure 7.57. – *Postero-anterior meta-carpophalangeal movement*

Method

The postero-anterior movement is produced by pressure acting through the tip of her right thumb against the posterior surface of the head of the proximal phalanx immediately adjacent to the metacarpophalangeal joint. The movement, which can be performed in any degree of meta-carpophalangeal flexion or extension, must not be produced by the flexors of the right thumb.

Anteroposterior movement***

Starting position

The physiotherapist grasps the patient's second metacarpal between her fully flexed left index finger anteriorly and the tip of her thumb which contacts the posterior surface of the metacarpal distally. She holds the proximal phalanx of his index finger between her fully flexed right finger and thumb, with her proximal interphalangeal joint against the anterior surface of the head of the proximal phalanx adjacent to the joint and her right thumb against the posterior surface of the phalanx more distally (*Figure 7.58*).

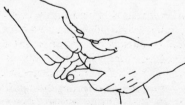

Figure 7.58. – *Anteroposterior metacarpophalangeal movement*

Method

The oscillation is produced by an anteroposterior pressure against the head of the proximal phalanx anteriorly. This movement may be performed in any degree of metacarpophalangeal flexion or extension.

When general mobilizing of all fingers in every direction is used as a general loosening procedure the following techniques may be used. These techniques are less specific but they have the effect of making the joints feel freer and more comfortable.

GENERAL FLEXION, EXTENSION, CIRCUMDUCTION

*Starting position**

The physiotherapist holds across the back of the patient's right hand from the medial side with her left hand. She grasps through his first interosseous space with her fingers to reach his palm and holds across the back of his hand with her thenar eminence and thumb. With her right hand she holds his four fingers, also from the medial side, between her fingers anteriorly and her thenar eminence posteriorly. With this grasp she can perform flexion, extension or circumduction.

Method

1. From a position of say 60 degrees of metacarpophalangeal flexion and almost full interphalangeal extension the physiotherapist can extend the metacarpophalangeal joints while at the same time flexing the interphalangeal joints. This movement can be performed as a grade II movement (*Figure 7.59a* and *b*). The reverse movement is then performed to reach the starting position.

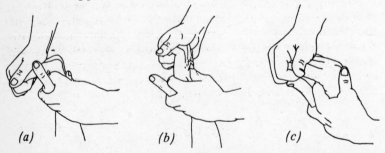

(a)   *(b)*   *(c)*

Figure 7.59. – General movements metacarpophalangeal and interphalangeal joints. (a) and (b) flexion/extension; (c) circumduction

2. With the middle and distal phalanges held firmly in her right hand she can carry out circumduction of the metacarpophalangeal joints by a circling action with her right hand. During all of these movements she must hold his metacarpals very firmly between the fingers and thumb of her left hand *(Figure 7.59c)*.

TREATMENT

The metacarpal and interphalangeal joints are so shaped that as the joint is flexed the distal joint surface 'slides' anteriorly on the proximal joint surface. It would seem therefore, at least theoretically, that if one of these joints is painlessly stiff in flexion then to stretch the joint structures by using grade IV flexion movements, pressure should be applied to the posterior surface of the base of the distal bone at the same time, to encourage that forward movement of the base on the head.

When flexion is painful as well as restricted then during the use of flexion as a stretching technique the base of the distal bone forming the joint should be moved anteroposteriorly as well as posteroanteriorly.

It is uncommon for a patient to have pain arising from one of these joints without some degree of stiffness. Under these circumstances all of the necessary movements (rotation, transverse movement both medially and laterally, anteroposterior and postero-anterior movements, distraction, abduction and adduction) should be utilized at the limit of the range. Following these stretching techniques the loosening movements shown in *Figure 7.59* should be carried out.

THUMB MOVEMENTS

Movements of the thumb are identical with those of the fingers even though the planes of the thumb movements do not coincide with those of the fingers. The movement of opposition is an additional thumb movement. Opposition takes place at the carpometacarpal joint and in terms of passive movement it is a combination of flexion, abduction, and rotation. Because the carpometacarpal joint lies in a different plane its movements will be described.

QUICK TESTS

Varying angles of postero-anterior pressure on the trapezium, trapezoid, base of first metacarpal and the joint line combined with extension are quick to perform and are usually very informative. Table 7.12 outlines the examination.

Table 7.12
Carpometacarpal Joint of Thumb: Objective Examination

[The routine examination of this joint must include the adjacent intercarpal joints and wrist]

Observation

Active movements
 Active quick tests as described for wrist joint
 Add active movements of thumb including gripping and fist

Static tests

Other structures in 'plan'
 Full active resisted movement through range for 'sheaths'
 Joint restriction c.f. muscle/tendon restriction

Passive movements
Physiological movements
 Routinely
  1. Wrist F, E, Ab, Ad
  2. Differentiating F, E, Ab and Ad
  3. Individual C/MC F, E, Ab, Ad
  4. HF and HE of carpus
  Note range, pain, resistance, spasm and behaviour
Accessory movements
 Routinely
  1. ↕ and ↕ of first metacarpal on trapezium
  2. →•→ and ←•← against metacarpal on carpus, with and without abduction and adduction, with and without compression
  3. ↻ and ↺ of metacarpal, with and without compression
  4. ↕ adjacent intercarpal and 1st C/MC joint
  Note range, pain, resistance, spasm and behaviour
 As applicable
  1. Intercarpal tests
  2. C/MC ↕ with E

Palpation
 Include tendon sheaths

Check case records etc.

HIGHLIGHT MAIN FINDINGS WITH ASTERISKS

After treatment

Flexion**

Starting position

The physiotherapist stabilizes the patient's wrist in her left hand with her fingers across the anterior surface and her thumb posteriorly. She must make sure that her index finger crosses in front of his trapezium

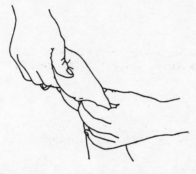

Figure 7.60. – Carpometacarpal flexion

to stabilize it during thumb flexion while not obstructing metacarpal movement. She grasps his thumb in her right hand with her thumb across the posterior surface of the metacarpal and her index finger across the anterior surface (*Figure 7.60*).

Method

The flexion movement is produced through her right hand while her left hand stabilizes the proximal part of the joint.

Extension**

Starting position

This is the same as that described above except that the tip of her left thumb is placed against the dorsal surface of the trapezium, with which the metacarpal articulates, and the trapezoid with which it has a ligamentous attachment (*Figure 7.61*).

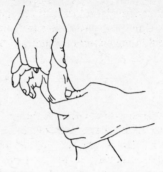

Figure 7.61. – Carpometacarpal extension

Method

The extension movement is produced mainly through her contact on the anterior surface of the first metacarpal pivoting it around her right thumb while her left thumb stabilizes the proximal part of the joint. The movements of flexion and extension can be performed in various degrees of abduction or adduction but the one usually used is the one which is most restricted or most painful.

Adduction, abduction and opposition***

Adduction, abduction and opposition are performed with basically the same techniques as described above. With one hand the physiotherapist stabilizes the carpus, particularly the trapezium, while the other hand produces the movement of the metacarpal in the desired direction. During opposition, medial rotation is included as part of the oscillatory movement.

Longitudinal movement cephalad***

This is produced by the same method as has already been described for the index finger (*see* page 194) and is used in treatment in much the same way. It can be used in conjunction with flexion, extension, abduction or adduction as dictated by the signs found on examination.

Postero-anterior movement

Pressures in postero-anterior, anteroposterior, medial and lateral directions can be exerted against the trapezium, the trapezoid or the base of
the first metacarpal. Only postero-anterior movement will be described
as the remainder should then be self-explanatory.

Starting position

The physiotherapist grasps the patient's thumb with her right hand
and the radial border of his wrist with her left hand. She places the
tips of both thumbs, tip to tip, in one of three main positions:
(1) against the posterior surface of the first metacarpal immediately
adjacent to the carpometacarpal joint (*Figure 7.62*); (2) against the
trapezium; or (3) on the joint line.

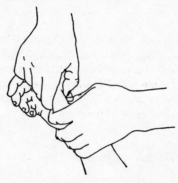

Figure 7.62. — Postero-anterior movement at the first carpometacarpal joint

Method

The postero-anterior movement is produced by pressure of the thumbs
against the base of the metacarpal. The pressure should arise from the
physiotherapist's arms and must not be produced by the thumb flexors.

TREATMENT

The carpometacarpal joints of the thumb are a common source of
pain. It is surprising how often the physiological movements of the

carpometacarpal joints of the thumb are painless both actively and passively yet when postero-anterior movement of the metacarpal on the trapezium, and/or when the joint surfaces are compressed during extension, the patient's symptoms are immediately reproduced. Use of this technique, interposing III− grades between stretching IV or IV+ grades with a controlled degree of pain, is dramatically effective.

8 Lower Limb

HIP JOINT

The hip is much more stable than the shoulder joint. Movement at the hip cannot be produced by thumb pressure against the head of the femur to the same degree as it can be produced in the glenohumeral joint. The shape of the acetabulum and the accessibility of the head of the femur make this impossible. However, small oscillatory movements of the head of the femur within the acetabulum can be produced particularly when the leg is used as a lever.

EXAMINATION

The routine examination for the hip joint is given in Table 8.1

QUICK TESTS

The quickest way to make a general assessment of the patient's hip disorder is to ask him to walk forwards in his usual manner and to walk backwards, then to flex his hip and knee so as to put his foot up on a step. If those movements do not reveal any abnormality he should be asked to squat, firstly allowing him to do it as he chooses and secondly observing any differences if he squats while on his toes or with his feet flat on the floor.

Table 8.1
Hip Joint: Objective Examination

Observation

Active movements
    Active quick tests
    Routinely
        Gait, squatting, (flexing knee to chest, going up step)
        Lumbar spine

Static tests

Other joints in 'plan'

Passive movements
Physiological movements
        1. F/Ad
          or
        F, E, ↻ and ↺ in F and E, Ab, and Ad, E

        2. Tensor fascia lata
        Note range, pain, resistance, spasm and behaviour

Accessory movements
    As applicable
        1. ↔ , ceph and caud ↕ , ↑ , →, ← (and ↻ ↺) in various
          hip positions
        2. Add compression where applicable

        Note range, pain, resistance, spasm and behaviour

Palpation

Check case records etc.

HIGHLIGHT MAIN FINDINGS WITH ASTERISKS

After treatment

SPECIAL TESTS

There is one particular combination movement which should be used as a test movement in an endeavour to elicit joint signs when other movements are normal. The test involves flexion/adduction through an arc from 90 to 140 degree flexion. This movement will be described first as it can be used as a quick method for testing normality of the joint.

Flexion/adduction

Flexion/adduction is as important to the hip as the quadrant movement is to the glenohumeral joint. While all other movements are pain free, this movement can be restricted and painful when compared with the opposite hip. Used as grade III or IV it is extremely useful when treating a hip which is the source of minor symptoms. Grade II type movements can be used effectively in the treatment of osteoarthritic hips during an exacerbation.

GRADE IV***

Starting position

The patient lies near the right-hand edge of the couch while the physiotherapist stands by his right thigh, facing across his body. She flexes his hip to a right angle allowing his knee to flex comfortably. She interlocks the fingers of both hands and cups them over the top of his knee. She then adducts his hip fully until his right ilium starts to lift from the couch. To maintain balance, she places her right knee on the couch, level with left knee, and leans against the lateral surface of his femur so that her chin is close to her hands. Her left thigh, pressed firmly against the edge of the couch at the level of his right hip, gives her the added control to prevent her weight falling fully against his right thigh (*Figure 8.1*).

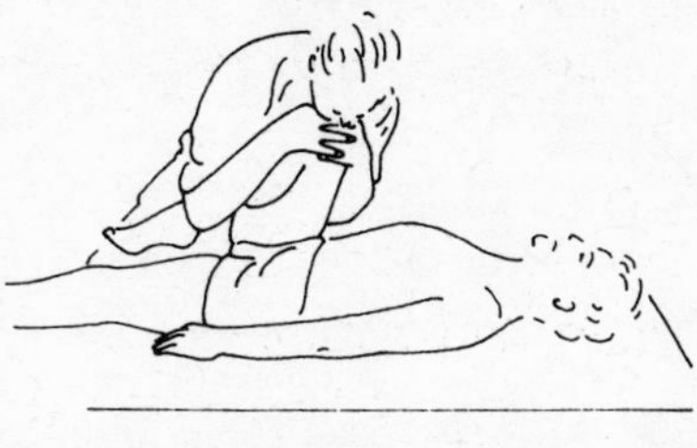

Figure 8.1. – Hip joint; flexion/adduction

Method

To find the position of the limitation which requires treatment, the hip should be moved through an arc of flexion in adduction from 90 degrees hip flexion to approximately 140 degrees where the knee is pointing towards the patient's left shoulder. To test this arc of movement the physiotherapist, starting with the patient's hip in a position of 90 degrees of flexion and full adduction, applies and maintains a constant pressure through the knee along the shaft of the femur in these two directions while at the same time moving his thigh through a further 50 degrees of flexion. At all times during the movement the femur should lie midway between medial and lateral rotation. When movement is normal the knee will follow the arc of a circle (*Figure 8.2a*). A small abnormality will be felt as a bump on the smooth arc of this circle (*Figure 8.2b*) and this point may be painful. The movement should always be compared with movement of the other hip.

Grade IV movements can be directed against the painful limitation in three ways. The first is simply a flexion/adduction movement directed at the limitation; this movement is depicted as a single-headed arrow in *Figure 8.2c*. The second method is to move from flexion through 10 or more degrees of extension and then to return while maintaining moderate

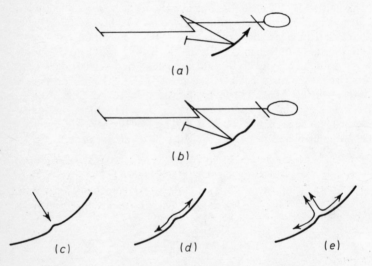

(a)

(b)

(c)   (d)   (e)

Figure 8.2. – Diagrammatic representation of hip flexion/adduction

pressure in adduction so that the movement can rub back and forth over the painful limitation. A double-headed arrow in *Figure 8.2d* depicts this movement. The third method, perhaps the most important of all, is the small movement which nudges at either side of the limitation in back and forth oscillations in an arc, as shown in *Figure 8.2e* by the two double-headed arrows.

TECHNIQUES

Flexion/adduction

GRADE III***

Starting position

The physiotherapist rests her right knee on the couch and leans her left thigh against the edge. Having flexed the patient's hip, she holds his flexed knee with her two hands and then adducts and flexes his hip to

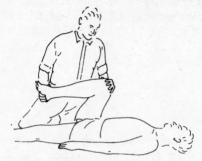

Figure 8.3. – Hip joint; flexion/adduction, grade III

the limit of the range at the chosen point on the arc. Before commencing the oscillatory movement she alters her grip to support his knee entirely with her left hand, leaving her right hand free to support his right foot and thus prevent flapping. In this position she maintains the mid-rotation movement (*Figure 8.3*).

Method

The large amplitude oscillation of approximately 30 degrees directed towards the limitation must traverse a straight line and the amplitude of foot movement must equal that of his knee. With her body positioned to form the stop at the outer limit of the movement, she swings his knee away from her to the limit of the flexion/adduction range where his pelvis begins to lift from the couch. These large amplitude oscillations are difficult to perform smoothly without hip rotation. They are, however, extremely valuable in the treatment of the moderately painful hip.

GRADE II***

Starting position

The physiotherapist stands at the level of the patient's right thigh, facing his left shoulder. After flexing his right hip and knee she positions her body as a stop at the lateral extent of the flexion/adduction movement. She holds his knee in her left hand and his foot in her right and

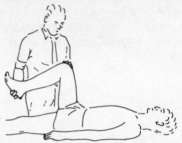

Figure 8.4. – Hip joint; flexion/adduction, grade II

faces in the direction of the flexion/adduction movement. She stands further away from the patient for this grade than for grade III (*Figure 8.4*).

Method

The 30 degree large amplitude movement, which does not reach the limit of the range, is performed by a back and forth movement of the physiotherapist's arms. The depth of range into which this is taken is governed by the onset of pain and whether this pain increases with further movement. This technique, in its various grades, is among the most useful of all hip mobilizations.

Neither flexion nor adduction will be described as separate techniques because they are simply variations of the foregoing, and also because they are not usually restricted when flexion/adduction is free.

Medial rotation

This movement, which is frequently restricted and painful, may be more restricted in hip flexion than in extension or vice versa, and such variations should be sought during examination. When movement is very painful, and grade I or II movements are required for treatment, they should be performed in the position as near to midway between the limits of normal physiological flexion and extension as comfort will permit. This is the position where movement is freest and in which a patient relaxes best.

Although the technique shown in *Figure 8.5* is titled rotation, it is related to rotation of the femur and not rotation, that is 'spin', of the hip joint.[1] In fact, when the femur rotates, the movement of the head of the femur in the acetabulum is a combination of 'slide' and 'roll' combined with a small degree of abduction and adduction. The abduction and adduction occur because when the physiotherapist rolls the patient's knee away from her, the posterior aspect of the patient's knee does not slide on the physiotherapist's thigh but adducts slightly. Similarly, as she pulls the knee back towards her, the knee moves laterally, that is, it adducts.

When grades III and IV are required, the movement should be performed in the degree of flexion or extension where the painful limitation exists or, if general mobilization is required, it should be performed in both flexion and extension.

GRADES I AND II***

Starting position

The patient lies near the right-hand edge of the couch. The physiotherapist stands at the level of his right knee. With her right knee on

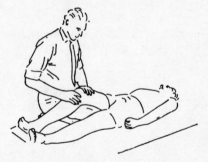

Figure 8.5. – Hip joint; medial rotation, grades I and II

the couch she positions her thigh carefully to support his thigh and calf to give him a comfortable and small degree of hip and knee flexion while his heel rests on the couch. She holds around his knee with both hands (*Figure 8.5*).

[1] *Gray's Anatomy* (1973), p. 405. 35th Edition. Edinburgh; Churchill Livingstone

Method

She imparts small rotary movements to the femur by light pressures against the lateral surface of his knee. For grade I movement very little movement should be performed whereas when grade II is required a large amplitude of medial rotation is performed.

ALTERNATIVE METHOD FOR GRADE I

Starting position

The patient lies on his left side with pillows between his legs so as to support his hip in a neutral and pain-free position. The physiotherapist leans across his hip, positioning it in her left axilla and with her left

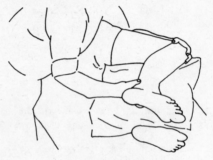

Figure 8.6. — Hip joint; medial rotation,
alternative method for grade I

hand she holds around and under his knee so as to stabilize it and to feel hip rotation. With her right hand she holds under his right ankle and foot to stabilize the foot.

Method

While the physiotherapist holds around the knee with her left hand, maintaining a constant position of abduction/adduction and flexion/ extension, she produces very small oscillatory movements by raising and lowering the patient's foot with her right hand.

Throughout the technique the patient should be questioned, to determine whether any pain or discomfort is felt in the hip.

IN EXTENSION SUPINE (GRADES III AND IV)**

Starting position

The patient lies supine near the right-hand edge of the couch on a slight angle to bring his left foot near the edge of the couch and leave his right knee free of the edge. The physiotherapist, kneeling by his right thigh, facing his left knee, supports under his knee with her left forearm, and holds his right foot with her right hand. While stabilizing his knee with her left forearm, she medially rotates his hip by raising his heel laterally (*Figure 8.7*).

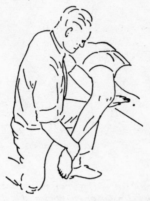

Figure 8.7. – Hip joint; medial rotation in extension supine, grades III and IV

Method

The physiotherapist produces grade IV movements by moving the patient's right foot laterally to the limit of the range while maintaining an equal and opposite counterpressure against the lateral side of his knee with her left forearm. Oscillatory rotation is controlled by her right hand. The pressure with her left arm should be quite firm; in fact this hand feels the tension of the movement even more than does her right hand.

When grade III movements are required, a large amplitude oscillation is produced by lowering the patient's right foot which releases the pressure against her left arm. While raising and lowering his foot she must exercise care maintaining the patient's thigh in a constant position so that only medial rotation is produced.

IN EXTENSION PRONE (GRADES III AND IV)**

Starting position

The patient lies prone and flexes his knee to a right angle. The physiotherapist, standing by his right knee, facing his hip, rests her left knee
on the couch, her thigh forming a comfortable stop for his leg at the

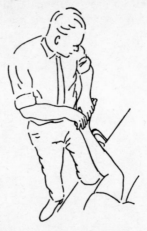

*Figure 8.8. – Hip joint; medial rotation
in extension prone, grades III and IV*

limit of medial rotation of his hip. She holds his heel in her right hand
and his forefoot in her left, medially rotating his hip and adjusting her
left leg to the height required to prevent further medial rotation
(*Figure 8.8*).

Method

The physiotherapist produces medial rotation of the patient's hip by
drawing his foot towards her until it reaches her thigh. The foot and leg
are then repeatedly oscillated back and forth by her arms. A better
action is usually obtained if, while she draws his foot towards her, she
inverts his foot a little. She may need to position her right hand against
the lateral side of his thigh during the medial rotation to prevent hip
abduction. Treatment movements from II+ to IV– can be given with
complete control in this position.

IN FLEXION (GRADES III AND IV)**

Starting position

The patient lies supine near the right-hand edge of the couch and the physiotherapist stands by his right hip, facing his left knee. She flexes his hip and knee to a right angle, supporting his knee with her left hand

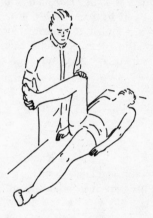

Figure 8.9. – Hip joint; medial rotation in flexion, grades III and IV

and his right heel with her right hand. She medially rotates his hip, preventing abduction by pressure against the lateral surface of his knee with her left hand (*Figure 8.9*).

Method

Medial rotation is produced by her right hand moving his foot in an arc around his knee while maintaining a constant knee position with her left hand.

Lateral rotation

Lateral rotation is rarely required. When necessary, it is usually performed with the hip in flexion. When the joint is painful, requiring grade I or II movements, the technique is identical with that described for medial rotation except for the direction of the movement (*Figure 8.5*). An alternative position for grade I is for the technique to be performed in exactly the same way as described for medial rotation with the patient lying on his left side and having pillows between his legs. The one difference is that the physiotherapist's right hand produces lateral rotation as very small oscillatory movements by gently pushing the patient's foot into the pillows and then returning it to its starting position. The position is as in *Figure 8.6* but with the difference that the physiotherapist's right hand holds around the foot and ankle. Grades III and IV are similar to those performed for medial rotation except that in extension the technique cannot easily be performed with the patient supine because the edge of the treatment couch hinders movement of the leg.

IN FLEXION SUPINE*

Starting position

The physiotherapist stands by the patient's right hip, facing his left knee, and flexes his hip and knee to a right angle. She holds his knee in her left hand and his foot in her right hand. Stabilizing his knee with her left hand, she laterally rotates his hip until the limit of the range is reached, at the same time adjusting the position of her body to face his left shoulder (*Figure 8.10*).

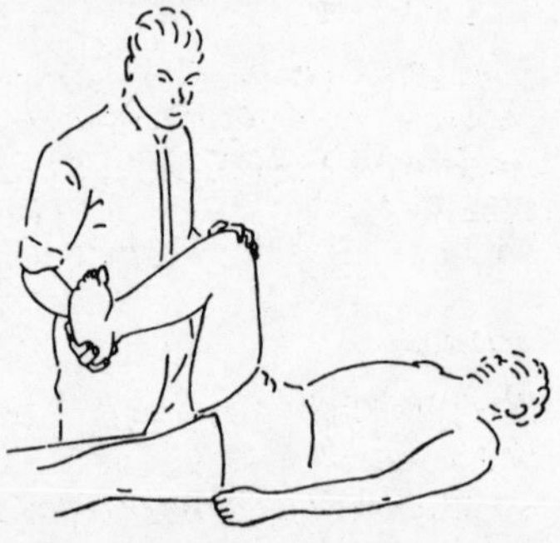

Figure 8.10. – *Hip joint; lateral rotation in flexion supine*

Method

Grade III or IV oscillatory movements are produced by moving the patient's foot back and forth in an arc around his knee. The physiotherapist's left hand and trunk maintain the position of his knee, the centre of the arc of movement. If the hip is flexed a few degrees during the medial rotation phase of the oscillation and then extended back through those few degrees during lateral rotation, the technique is sometimes easier. This action lessens the amount of work for the right hand.

IN EXTENSION PRONE*

Starting position

The patient lies prone and the physiotherapist stands by his left knee, facing his right hip. She flexes his right knee to a right angle, holds his right forefoot with her right hand and his heel with her left hand. With

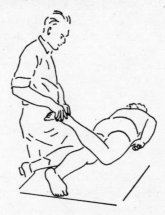

Figure 8.11. – Hip joint; lateral rotation in extension prone

her right knee on the couch, she positions her thigh to provide the stop at the limit of his lateral rotation. She then laterally rotates his hip by lowering his foot towards her until the limit of the range is reached (*Figure 8.11*).

Method

The physiotherapist performs the oscillatory rotation by a back and forth action with her arms. The technique is improved if the lateral rotation movement is combined with some eversion of his foot.

Lateral movement**

This movement is depicted with the hip positioned in almost 90 degrees of flexion. It must be realized, however, that exactly the same lateral movement of the hip can be produced in any degree of hip flexion or extension, in different angles of abduction or adduction, and with varying degrees of rotation.

Starting position

The patient lies on his back and flexes his hip and knees to the chosen angle. The physiotherapist stands alongside the patient's hip, pressing her upper sternum against his knee while interlocking her fingers and holding around the medial surface of his thigh as near as is practicable to the hip joint. Her arms and chest also stabilize his lower leg (*Figure 8.12*).

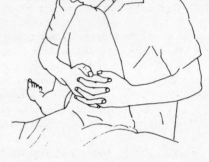

Figure 8.12. – Hip joint; lateral movement

Method

Considerable movement can be produced by this technique. It can be used solely as a lateral displacement of the head of the femur in the acetabulum. To achieve this movement the physiotherapist should ensure that the angle of hip abduction or adduction does not alter as the proximal end of the femur is moved laterally. This may require considerable movement of the patient's knee position to avoid the tendency of his pelvis to roll as the hands pull the head of the femur laterally. Again, it is not the physiotherapist's hands which produce the lateral oscillatory movement. This time the patient's whole limb and the physiotherapist's hands, arms and thorax move as one solid entity while she rocks back and forth on her feet. By this method she can produce any movement between grade I and IV.

Alternatively, while producing the lateral movement of the hip joint, the physiotherapist may

1. stabilize the patient's knee, preventing its lateral movement, so that the lateral movement of the hip is combined with a small degree of horizontal adduction of the hip; or
2. while stabilizing the patient's limb and applying lateral movement to the hip, lean backwards, carrying the patient's hip into a small degree of horizontal abduction.

If the technique is to be used as an accessory movement at the limit of another range of movement as part of the treatment to restore range, then before applying lateral movement she should position the hip at the limit of the range she aims to improve (i.e. the limit of flexion, extension, abduction, adduction, medial rotation or lateral rotation) before taking up any remaining slack in the direction of lateral movement. She should then use the oscillatory lateral movement as a grade IV or IV+ movement. Also, under circumstances where improvement in range is the goal, the lateral movement asserted by the physiotherapist's hands may be performed simultaneously with movement in the direction of the chosen upper range. For example if the aim is to improve medial rotation the starting position is adopted where the hip is flexed to a neutral convenient position and medially rotated to the limit of the range. To perform the technique the physiotherapist twists her trunk to face towards his feet while producing the lateral movement. Again it is emphasized that the patient's whole limb and the physiotherapist's hands, arms and trunk move as one entity as movement is produced by the rocking action on her feet.

When extremely gentle and very finely controlled lateral movement is needed a different starting position must be used.

GRADE I**

Starting position

The patient lies on his side and pillows are placed between his comfortably flexed legs. The physiotherapist stands behind the patient and grasps around his thigh anteriorly and superiorly (*Figure 8.13*).

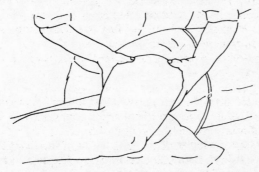

Figure 8.13. — Hip joint; lateral movement, grade I

Method

The physiotherapist very gently oscillates a lateral hip movement. She should endeavour, with the whole palmar surfaces of her fingers, to feel the femur and control the tiny movements. It is also necessary repeatedly to determine by questioning if the movement is free of pain.

Longitudinal movement caudad***

Longitudinal movement is most useful when hip movements are very painful. The amount of movement possible is very small but when the patient has considerable pain and it is performed in a comfortable position for the patient this movement is soothing.

Starting position

The physiotherapist supports under the patient's slightly flexed hip and knee with her right leg. Depending upon the amount of hip flexion which is comfortable for the patient, she either kneels on her right shin and places her right thigh diagonally under his knee, or she sits on the

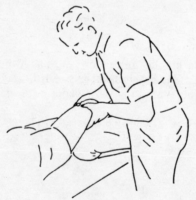

*Figure 8.14. – Hip joint; longitudinal
movement caudad*

edge of the couch and places her right leg fully flexed at the knee and laterally rotated at the hip, under his thigh. She then encircles the distal end of his femur with her hands (*Figure 8.14*).

Method

Oscillatory longitudinal movements are produced by pulling gently on the femur. This technique can be assisted by a rolling or sliding movement of the physiotherapist's support under the patient's thigh in the direction of the treatment movement. When the joint is very painful, movements should be performed so gently that there is no discomfort. This technique can be performed in varying degrees of hip flexion.

ALTERNATIVE METHOD FOR GRADE I

Starting position

The patient lies on his left side with the pillows between his legs. His hips are positioned in mid flexion/extension and his knees comfortably flexed. The physiotherapist, standing behind the patient, places her

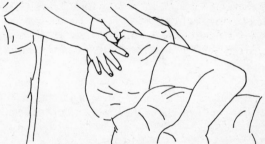

Figure 8.15. – Hip joint; longitudinal movement caudad, alternative method for grade I

thumbs on the greater trochanter, her fingers spread widely to help stabilize the thumb position, and her forearms directed in line with the patient's femur (*Figure 8.15*).

Method

Extremely gentle comfortable longitudinal movements can be produced at the hip joint by this method. It is important that the thumbs should not be the prime movers in producing the oscillatory movement but should act as spring-like contact points, feeling the movement which is taking place. The physiotherapist's arm and body gently rock back and forth in line with the femur to produce the hip movement.

ALTERNATIVE METHOD FOR GRADE I OR II**

Starting position

The patient lies on his left side with pillows between his legs to limit adduction of the right hip. The patient's hips and knees are flexed for comfort and for positioning the hip in a neutral position.

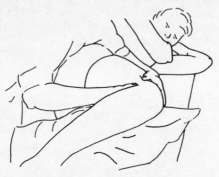

Figure 8.16. – Hip joint; Longitudinal movement caudad, alternative method for grade I or II

The physiotherapist leans across the patient, cradling his pelvis with her left axilla. She then grasps the lower end of the femur with both hands (*Figure 8.16*).

Method

The physiotherapist stabilizes the pelvis in her left axilla to prevent it moving while the technique is being performed. The longitudinal movement is produced through her hands, which clasp the distal end of the femur. The movement should be produced by her arms; she cannot use her body because she would then lose control of the patient's pelvis position.

IN FLEXION

Longitudinal movement of the hip is an accessory movement which can be used with the femur in many different positions. The two following techniques show longitudinal movement being applied to the hip while it is in flexion. The first is neither adducted nor abducted during the technique and the second, while still in flexion, is also in some degree of abduction.

Starting position (in flexion)

The patient's hip is flexed to 90 degrees and his knee is fully flexed. The physiotherapist, with the fingers of both hands interlocked, grasps

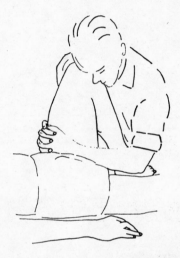

Figure 8.17. – Hip joint; longitudinal movement caudad in flexion

around the anterior surface of his thigh as far proximally as she can reach. She stabilizes the hip and knee angle by cradling his knee between her head and shoulder (*Figure 8.17*).

Method (in flexion)

The physiotherapist's grasp of the patient's leg is such that, as she rocks back and forth on her feet, her whole trunk and the patient's leg rock in the same direction.

Starting position (in flexion/abduction)

The starting position for this technique is identical with that described for the preceding technique except that the patient's femur is abducted to any chosen range (*Figure 8.18*).

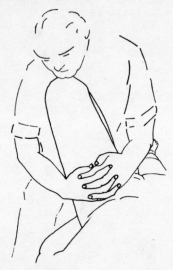

Figure 8.18. – Hip joint; longitudinal movement caudad in flexion/abduction

Method (in flexion/abduction)

The method used for producing the longitudinal movement is identical with that described for the preceding technique. The patient's leg and the physiotherapist's trunk and arms move as a single unit as she rocks back and forth on her feet.

Longitudinal movement cephalad***

The compression technique can be used on its own or in conjunction with rotation in the gentle grades, or with flexion and extension when these movements are performed between full extension and 20 degrees of flexion. It is best suited to the patient who has pain on weight bearing. It therefore serves its best purpose in grades III and IV.

Starting position

The physiotherapist supports the patient's leg in a slight degree of hip and knee flexion in the same way as described above for longitudinal movement caudad. She holds his leg with her right hand cupped over the tibial tubercle while supporting under his knee with her left hand (*Figure 8.19*).

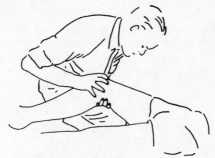

Figure 8.19. – Hip joint; longitudinal movement cephalad

Method

The oscillatory movement, pushing the head of the femur into the acetabulum, is performed by the physiotherapist's right hand thrusting against the front of the tibia in the line of the femur. The return oscillation is governed almost entirely by her left hand. As with the caudad technique the movement can be performed in varying degrees of hip flexion. If strong techniques are used there will be considerable pelvic movement. The strength of technique is varied either to produce slight pain or to reach a point just short of this.

Postero-anterior movement**

Very little postero-anterior movement of the head of the femur takes place in the acetabulum. However, this technique can be used to good effect for the very painful joint. It can also be used as an accessory movement at the limit of a physiological range when the aim of treatment is to increase the range of movement of the hip joint.

When used for treating pain, pillows are used and the thigh is positioned midway between the limit of its ranges. Usually this means that the hip is flexed, the correct range being that which is pain free. Very gentle oscillatory movements which are painless should be produced by thumb pressures.

When the movements are being used to increase the range of movement in any particular direction, flexion for example, the hip is flexed to the limit of its range and the physiotherapist's hands rather than her thumbs are used to produce the postero-anterior movement.

Starting position

The patient lies on his left side with pillows between his legs and thighs. The physiotherapist stands behind him and places the pads of both thumbs, pointing towards each other, against the posterior surface of the greater trochanter (*Figure 8.20*). This is the starting position for grades I and II.

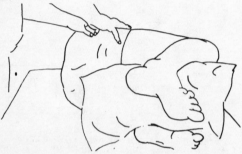

Figure 8.20. – Hip joint; postero-anterior movement

If the technique is being used as a stretching technique, the patient's hip is flexed as far as possible and the physiotherapist applies the oscillatory grade IV movement, using the heel of her hand.

Method

When painless grade I movements are used for treating pain, soft gentle small amplitude oscillatory movements are produced by the physiotherapist's body and arms through the thumbs stabilized against the trochanter. As with other techniques which make use of the physiotherapist's thumbs, the movement should not be produced by the thumb's intrinsic muscles. Throughout the technique the patient is asked if he can feel any pain or discomfort.

When the technique is used for stretching hip flexion the physiotherapist may need to use one hand against the femur while the other hand maintains hip flexion and/or stabilizes the pelvis by pressure anteroposteriorly against the right anterosuperior iliac spine.

Anteroposterior movement

Starting position

The patient lies on his left side with pillows between his legs and thighs as described above. The physiotherapist stands in front of the patient and places her thumbs on the anterior surface of the greater trochanter. She should endeavour to use a large surface area of the pads of the thumbs so as to make the technique as comfortable as possible. Spreading her fingers will help to stabilize her thumbs, which should be in direct bone-to-bone contact with the trochanter (*Figure 8.21*).

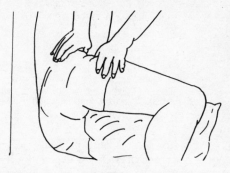

Figure 8.21. – Hip joint; anteroposterior movement

Method

As described above the oscillatory movement is produced by the physiotherapist's body and arms and not by intrinsic thumb muscles.

Although the movement has been described as, and titled, antero-posterior movement, the actual direction of the pressure against the anterior surface of the greater trochanter may be varied through an arc of approximately 30 degrees. If the technique is performed well it is surprising how much movement can be produced and felt.

Abduction

Abduction can be performed in three main ways. The first two are abduction in flexion and abduction in extension; the third is a combined extension/abduction movement which is the opposite from flexion/adduction described on page 207.

IN FLEXION*

It is simpler if abduction in flexion is performed in a position of approximately 60 degrees flexion with the patient's foot resting on the couch even though a degree of lateral rotation occurs with the abduction. Grades II and IV are the most frequently used treatment movements in

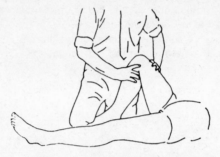

Figure 8.22. – Hip joint; abduction in flexion

this position. When the joint is very painful, grade I movements are used in a position of approximately 20 degrees hip flexion (*see Figure 8.14*). When grade IV movements are used, as in *Figure 8.22*, both legs should be flexed so that the painless hip can be abducted fully to stabilize the pelvis during the mobilization of the painful stiff hip.

Starting position

The physiotherapist stands by the flexed hip and knee of the patient, whose foot rests on the couch level with his left knee. She rests her right lower leg across his foot to stabilize it. She supports his knee with her left hand over the femur and her right hand over the tibia. Before performing the mobilization, she abducts his knee to the limit of the range which she intends using for treatment and stands close to his leg to form a stop, preventing further abduction (*Figure 8.22*).

Method

The oscillation is performed in small or large amplitudes by the action of her hands on his knee. His pelvis must be watched carefully to see that the hip movement is not taken beyond the point at which it begins to move.

IN EXTENSION**

The patient lies with both legs abducted comfortably. The physio-therapist, standing by his right lower leg, facing his hip, places her right knee immediately adjacent to his right leg. Sitting back on her right heel she supports under his right knee with her left hand and under his ankle with her right hand (*Figure 8.23*).

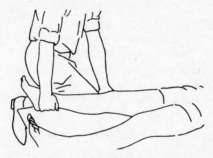

Figure 8.23. – Hip joint; abduction in extension

Method

The oscillation, usually not exceeding an amplitude of 10–15 degrees, is performed by the physiotherapist's arms while the patient's leg is supported just free of the couch. Her right leg forms the stop at the limit of the abduction range. If more hip extension is required, a folded blanket or pillow can be placed under the patient's buttocks.

Extension/abduction**

The main use for extension/abduction is to treat pain rather than to restore range by stretching. It is therefore used mainly as a grade II movement.

Starting position

The physiotherapist stands in a similar position to that described for flexion/adduction as a grade II movement (*see* page 207). The difference is that she moves backward to lower the patient's leg in extension/abduction to the limit of the treatment range.

Method

The mobilization is performed through an amplitude of 20—40 degrees of hip movement by the physiotherapist's arms while at the same time she carefully maintains the hip in a mid-rotation position.

Extension**

Extension is best performed with the patient supine because movement at the hip can be performed in any part of the range whether it is limited or not. If there is a limitation of extension, the physiotherapist supports under the patient's knee with her right thigh in much the same way as has been described for longitudinal movement (*see Figure 8.14,* page 218). The technique described here will be for a grade II movement.

Starting position

The patient lies near the right-hand edge of the couch and the physiotherapist stands by his right lower leg facing his left knee. She holds laterally around and under his knee with her left hand and under his heel from the medial side with her right hand (*Figure 8.24*).

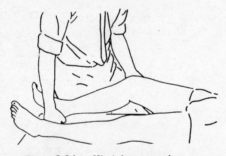

Figure 8.24. — Hip joint; extension

Method

The physiotherapist with her left hand raises his knee 6 or 8 inches from the couch and with her right hand keeps his heel off the couch and approximates it 3 or 4 inches towards his right buttock. She then carries his heel away from his buttock and allows his knee to lower to the limit of the extension. His heel is kept off the couch throughout the movement.

As has been mentioned, if the extension is limited she will support under his knee with her thigh to provide a stop at the limit of the movement. If a greater range of extension is required, a pillow can be placed under his buttocks. His left hip and knee may be flexed for comfort.

TREATMENT

The majority of patients referred for physiotherapy to the hip have, on examination of hip movements, a combination of stiffness and pain. It then becomes a question of priorities: should the physiotherapist initially treat pain or restriction of movement? It is usually wiser to treat pain for at least the first one or two sessions. If treating pain does not effect improvement, the stiffness can be treated and the only loss to the patient will have been time. However, if the choice is made to treat stiffness first and it causes a marked exacerbation then although it will not harm the joint disorder it does produce unnecessary discomfort for the patient, and it shows that the wrong approach was used at the current phase of the disorder.

The rotary technique shown in *Figure 8.5* (page 209) is very useful for the treatment of hip pain. Earlier in this book emphasis was placed on using accessory joint movements in a neutral position when techniques are directed towards treating the pain. Although this rotary technique is not an accessory movement, it is of particular value in the treatment of pain when a patient has a diagnosis of osteoarthritis of the hip. It is also most useful to relieve soreness when this soreness is produced by strong stretching techniques.

Another technique of great value is flexion/adduction. The technique, in its different grades, has been described in detail in this chapter. If a patient has minimal pain, or intermittent pain provoked by sudden unexpected movements, then flexion/adduction performed as a grade IV movement readily relieves this pain. This treatment technique would be performed as shown in *Figure 8.2c, d* and *e* (page 206). Obviously, the technique will cause discomfort or pain but this pain is readily relieved by performing the technique as shown in *Figure 8.2c* as a very gentle but large amplitude grade III movement.

When the hip joint is stiff, restricting functional activities, the same pattern of treatment is used as has been described in Chapter 5. That is, the particular movement which is restricted is performed as a gentle grade IV oscillatory movement for one minute or so, and is followed by grade III accessory movements at the limit of the restricted range.

This routine is repeated three or four times. Any treatment soreness is then easily relieved by performing a large painless grade III movement in the direction of the stiff movement being stretched.

KNEE

The techniques will be divided into those applied to the tibiofemoral joint and the patellofemoral articulation.

TIBIOFEMORAL JOINT

The tibiofemoral joint, like the elbow, has physiological movements of flexion and extension, and accessory movements of abduction, adduction, rotation, postero-anterior and anteroposterior movements, medial and lateral movements, longitudinal movement and compression.

EXAMINATION

QUICK TESTS

A variety of tests can be used to assess the severity of a patient's knee disorder, and a particular sequence of tests is suggested below. If test 2 reveals obvious pain and restriction of joint range then there is no need to proceed with tests 3 and 4. However, if test 2 does not give the information being sought then tests 3 and 4 can be usefully used. The range of knee movement may be measured and the degree and site of pain provoked by these tests can be recorded and used as asterisked signs against which progress can be measured. The tests are as follows.

1. The patient, sufficiently undressed, should be asked to walk forward away from the physiotherapist and to return while she assesses any abnormality or asymmetry in his gait.

   If the gait seems normal and symmetrical then the patient should be asked to walk backwards away from and towards the physiotherapist. This often reveals asymmetry in gait not seen when walking forward.

2. The patient should be asked to squat, using his hands to maintain balance if necessary. He should not be told to squat in any particular manner. The physiotherapist observes the spontaneous method he uses. It is his knee for which the quick tests are

being used so it matters little whether he squats with his feet flat or on his toes.

If he is able to do so, he should be asked to bounce in the full squat position, vigorously enough and with feet far enough apart, to bounce his buttocks downwards so that, if possible, his ischial tuberosities will pass his heels. The physiotherapist should make an assessment of any pain or discomfort; this is particularly important when the patient is able to bounce symmetrically. If the knee is normal the feeling in the joint which the patient experiences should be the same in both knees.

If the patient is only able to squat symmetrically a small distance and then continues to bend further by tilting towards the good side, the range of knee flexion on that side moves further while the painful side does not increase its range. Accordingly the physiotherapist should assess the range of knee flexion of the disordered knee together with the site and severity of pain.

3. It is useful to compare the range of knee flexion found in test 2 above with that which the patient can perform in the non-weight-bearing position lying supine.

4. Another useful test of knee flexion is to ask the patient to adopt the position where he is kneeling with his weight forwards on his hands. He should then be asked to sit back gradually until he reaches the limit of his range. If his range is normal he should be able to sit at least on his heels or even past his heels.

Tests 3 and 4 above are not strictly 'quick tests'. All of the information which the 'quick test' will give will be disclosed by tests 1 and 2. However, if test 2 reveals a marked limitation due either to joint stiffness or pain then tests 3 and 4 should follow logically so that the pattern of knee flexion is more clearly shown. It will be revealed more clearly because the test movements are done with the patient's full control and there will be no bodyweight transmitted through the joint.

SPECIAL TESTS

As has been mentioned in relation to other joints, the knee can be responsible for minor symptoms yet have a full painless range of flexion and extension. However, if grade IV extension/abduction, extension/adduction, flexion/abduction and flexion/adduction are not examined, the joint may be considered to be normal because important physical joint signs and reproduction of pain will have been missed. The two extension movements are the main test and extension/ abduction is the most common to elicit joint signs. These four movements are described under the heading 'Techniques'.

Table 8.2 below lists the full examination for the tibiofemoral joint.

Table 8.2
Tibiofemoral Joint: Objective Examination

[The routine examination of the tibiofemoral joint must also include examination of the patellofemoral (P/F) joint]

Observation

Active movements
    Active quick tests
  Routinely
    Gait, squatting
    Lumbar spine
  As applicable
    F and E in standing
    Specific movements which aggravate
    The injuring movement
    Movements under load
    Knee extension lag
    Speed of test movements

Static tests

Other joints in 'plan'

Passive movements
Physiological movements
  Routinely

    F, E, ↻ ↺ in F and E

    Note range, pain, resistance, spasm and behaviour
Accessory movements
  Routinely

    Ab, Ad, ↕ , ↑ , —••, ••— ,
As applicable
    E/Ab, E/Ad, F/Ab, F/Ad

    Note range, pain, resistance, spasm and behaviour

Palpation

Check case records etc.

HIGHLIGHT MAIN FINDINGS WITH ASTERISKS

After treatment

TECHNIQUES

Extension/abduction***

GRADE III

Starting position

The physiotherapist stands by the patient's right ankle, facing his left hip. She rests her right knee and lower leg on the couch at right angles to his leg and supports his right heel across her thigh adjacent to her anterior superior iliac spine. Her right hand supports his knee by being

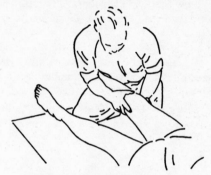

Figure 8.25. – Tibiofemoral extension/ abduction

placed around the medial aspect of the joint line so that her fingers reach the medial condyle of the tibia posteromedially and her thenar eminence covers it anteromedially. The heel of her left hand may be placed in one of three positions: cupped over the lateral epicondyle of the femur, on the lateral condyle of the tibia, or directly over the joint line. As with her right hand, the fingers of her left hand reach posteriorly while the thenar eminence is positioned slightly anteriorly. It is necessary for her left forearm to be almost at right angles to the shaft of the femur and tibia so that the abduction component can be produced (*Figure 8.25*).

Method

If a grade III movement is required, the patient's knee is raised and lowered through a distance of approximately 5 or 6 inches by the physiotherapist's hands. A constant pressure is maintained against the lateral surface of his knee by the heel of her left hand, placed in one of the three positions described above. Each of the three positions will produce a slightly different movement of the tibiofemoral joint. When the heel of her left hand is against the femur and a strong abducting pressure is applied, the femur will tend to move slightly medially on the tibia while abduction during extension is taking place at the joint. However, when the heel of her hand is placed against the tibia, the tibia will tend to move medially on the femur during the extension/abduction. When the heel of the physiotherapist's left hand is on the joint line there will be no medial movement of the femur on the tibia or tibia on the femur, so that the movement produced at the tibiofemoral joint will be simply extension/abduction. The stronger the abduction pressure required, the more she needs to crouch to bring her left shoulder close to his knee.

She must not support his lower leg above his ankle and she must firmly hold his foot against the iliac crest with her right elbow. This hold of his ankle enables the addition of longitudinal movement to the extension/abduction whenever it is required, as well as providing a counterpressure for the abduction pressure applied to the knee.

GRADE IV**

If grade IV+ movements are required, it is more economical for the physiotherapist to stand by the patient's right knee, holding from the lateral side under his heel with her right hand while her left hand is

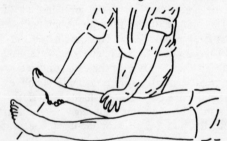

Figure 8.26. – Tibiofemoral extension/abduction, grade IV+

placed anterolaterally over the joint line of his knee. She is then in the best position to control firm small amplitude movements while varying the pressure of abduction or extension which she wishes to emphasize (*Figure 8.26*).

Extension/adduction***

The technique for extension/adduction is essentially the same as the technique described for grade III and IV+ extension/abduction, with the obvious difference that this time it is the physiotherapist's right forearm which should be at right angles to the femur and tibia so as to exert the adduction component. As described above for extension/abduction, the heel of her right hand can be placed over the medial epicondyle of the femur, the medial condyle of the tibia or the joint line. Also, as mentioned above, the three different positions of the heel of the physiotherapist's right hand produce three slightly different movements at the tibiofemoral joint.

Extension**

Sometimes the movement of extension is performed more effectively if the physiotherapist stablizes the patient's knee and produces extension by lifting his foot, rather than by using the technique described above which stabilizes the foot and lowers the knee. This may be because the techniques have slightly different tibiofemoral relationships and the patient may find it easier to relax with one than with the other.

Starting position

The physiotherapist stands by the patient's right thigh and kneels on her left shin to support under the lower end of his femur with her left thigh. When his knee is flexed and his foot supported on the couch, she moves her left thigh to his calf also. With both hands she holds distally around his lower leg from behind. Her left elbow should be by the inside of the patient's knee so that the axis of her left arm will coincide with the axis of his knee movement (*Figure 8.27*).

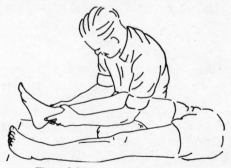

Figure 8.27. – Tibiofemoral extension

Method

This position is used for grade III movements and the amplitude is usually 25–30 degrees. The physiotherapist raises and lowers his leg through the arc of movement with her arms. An abduction or adduction component can be added to this movement if desired but the technique is less effective than that described previously (*see* page 233) where the three hand positions can be used.

Flexion/abduction***

Starting position

The physiotherapist, standing beside the patient's right knee, flexes his hip to a right angle and fully flexes his knee. She supports his knee in her left hand and grasps anteriorly around his ankle with her right hand

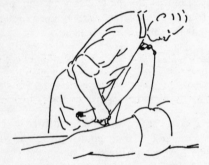

Figure 8.28. – Tibiofemoral flexion/abduction

so that with her fingers pushing laterally against the medial surface of his calcaneum posteriorly and her thumb hooked around his lateral malleolus she can fully medially rotate his tibia (*Figure 8.28*).

Method

This technique utilizes small or large amplitude oscillations as diagonal movements into flexion/abduction while strongly maintaining the rotation. His heel should be lateral to his ischial tuberosity. If the tibial rotation is lost the diagonal component of the movement will include medial rotation of the hip rather than the small abduction movement of the knee which can be produced. The physiotherapist needs to keep close to the patient's lower leg to enable her to control the pressure against the ankle.

Flexion/adduction***

Flexion/adduction is identical with that described above except that strong lateral rotation of the tibia is maintained throughout the diagonal movement of flexion/adduction. The starting position for the physiotherapist's right hand must be changed so that her fingers hook around

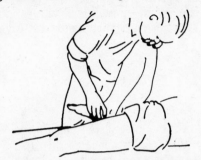

Figure 8.29. – Tibiofemoral flexion/adduction

the patient's medial malleolus while her thumb and the metacarpophalangeal joint of the index finger apply pressure in a posterior direction on the anterior surface of the tibia. Because of the adduction component, the patient's heel is directed medial to his ischial tuberosity (*Figure 8.29*).

Abduction and adduction**

The maximum amplitude of movement which can be produced in this direction is obtained when the knee is held approximately 10 degrees short of full extension.

Starting position

When this technique is used as a form of treatment, the position adopted is identical with that described for extension/abduction (*see* page 233). The physiotherapist maintains 10 degrees flexion by her finger support under the patient's knee (*see Figure 8.25*, page 233).

Method

Abduction movement is produced by the pressure of her left hand against the lateral surface of his knee. Adduction is produced by pressure against the medial side of his knee with her right hand.

Anteroposterior movement

The anteroposterior movement is very useful in the treatment of extremely painful knees when it is applied as a grade I movement with the knee supported on a soft pillow in a few degrees of flexion. In less painful conditions it can be used as a grade III or IV movement in any position of knee flexion. Anteroposterior movement has its greatest range in positions of knee flexion varying from 10 to 70 degrees.

GRADE I***

Starting position

The patient lies with a soft pillow placed under his knee, supporting the femur more than the tibia, in not more than 10 degrees of knee flexion. The physiotherapist stands by his right lower leg, facing his knee, and places the pads of her thumbs against the anterior surface of the tibia either side of the tibial tubercle. Her fingers rest against the adjacent surfaces of the tibia and fibula. She should position the metacarpophalangeal joints of her thumbs almost vertically above the pads so that the pressure will be directed through these joints (*Figure 8.30*).

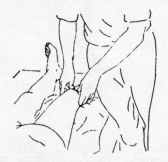

Figure 8.30. — Tibiofemoral anteroposterior movement, grade I

Method

Small oscillatory movements are produced by the physiotherapist's arms acting through her thumbs. These finely controlled movements should not be performed by the flexor muscles of the thumbs.

IN FLEXION (GRADE IV)***

Starting position

The patient lies with his foot resting on the couch so that his knee is is flexed approximately 70 degrees. The physiotherapist stands by his right ankle and rests her right lower leg across his foot to stabilize the

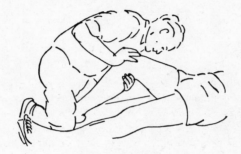

Figure 8.31. — Tibiofemoral antero-posterior movement, grade IV

position. She positions the heel of her right hand over the anterior surface of the tibia immediately adjacent to the joint line and spreads her fingers over the front of his knee. Her left hand is placed behind his knee with her palm over the upper calf (*Figure 8.31*).

Method

Anteroposterior mobilizing is produced by pressure of the heel of the physiotherapist's right hand against the upper end of the tibia. Her left hand acts as a support and produces the return movement when a large amplitude is required.

Postero-anterior movement**

Postero-anterior movements in grades I and IV have the same application in treatment as the anteroposterior movements and the techniques are essentially the same as those described above.

GRADE I

Starting position

For grade I movements the patient's knee is supported as shown in *Figure 8.32.*

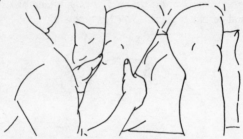

Figure 8.32. – *Tibiofemoral postero-anterior movement, grade I*

Method

The postero-anterior movement is produced by the physiotherapist's pressure transmitted through her fingers against the posterior surface of the tibia proximally.

GRADE IV

Starting position

For grade IV movements with the patient lying prone the physiotherapist rests her right tibia on the couch with her knee fully flexed while supporting the patient's distal shin across her upper thigh.

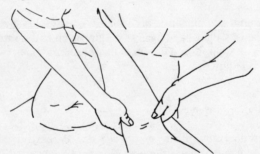

Figure 8.33. – *Tibiofemoral postero-anterior movement, grade IV*

There are two methods by which the movement can be produced. The physiotherapist can place the pads of her two thumbs on the posterior surfaces of the medial and lateral condyles of the tibia, using as much as possible of the pads of her thumbs, as bone-to-bone contact may be uncomfortable (*Figure 8.33*). Alternatively, she can support the patient's left shin in her right hand while the heel of her left hand is placed on the posterior surface of the tibia as far proximally as possible. The fingers of her left hand lie over the gastrocnemius (*Figure 8.34*).

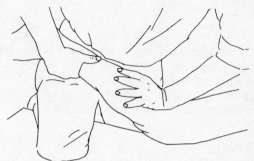

Figure 8.34. – Tibiofemoral postero-anterior movement, grade IV alternative position

Method

The grade IV oscillatory movements of the head of the tibia on the femur with the knee in some flexion, if performed by the thumbs, are produced by arm movement. In no circumstance should the oscillation be produced by the intrinsic thumb muscles because if this is done, the technique causes discomfort to the patient and the physiotherapist is unable to appreciate the extent and feel of the movement.

When the heel of the physiotherapist's left hand is used to produce the movement the pressure against the tibia originates from the physiotherapist's trunk and arm movement.

With this particular technique the movement can be performed in three slightly different ways, producing three distinctly different movements at the tibiofemoral joint.

1. As the head of the tibia is moved forwards the physiotherapist can, with her right hand, carry the distal end of the tibia an equal distance so that the whole lower leg moves through a full parallel line.

2. As the pressure is exerted postero-anteriorly through her left hand the physiotherapist can slightly lift the patient's distal tibia so that, combined with the anteroposterior movement, there will be a degree of knee flexion taking place.

3. As the postero-anterior movement at the head of the tibia is taking place the physiotherapist, with her right hand, can lower the distal end of the patient's tibia so that there is a degree of tibiofemoral extension as the postero-anterior movement is taking place.

Lateral movement**

Both lateral movement and medial movement (description of which follows this technique) are accessory movements and can be tested in various angles of knee flexion/extension. In the text which follows the knee is supported in a position of 90 degrees of flexion. The movement is described as movement of the tibia on the femur.

Starting position

With the patient lying supine, his hip and knee flexed and his foot resting on the table, the physiotherapist stands level with his foot and faces towards his head. She places the heel of her right hand on the medial condyle of the tibia and the heel of her left hand on the lateral epicondylar area of the femur. She then leans forwards and extends her wrists so that both forearms are directed parallel to each other. Her right forearm will be positioned on a slightly lower plane than her left forearm (*Figure 8.35*).

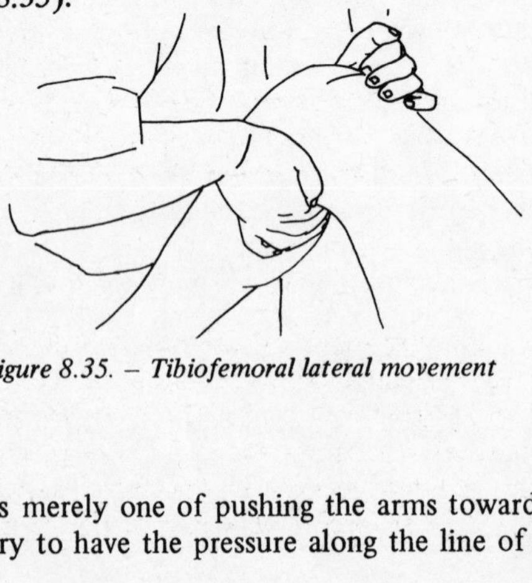

Figure 8.35. – Tibiofemoral lateral movement

Method

The technique is merely one of pushing the arms towards each other, but it is necessary to have the pressure along the line of each forearm directed correctly such that if the patient's knee were not there the physiotherapist's right arm would pass parallel to but below her left arm.

Medial movement**

Starting position

The difference in position between medial movement and lateral movement is that the physiotherapist changes her contact points around the patient's knee. For medial movement she places the heel

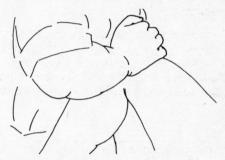

Figure 8.36. – Tibiofemoral medial movement

of her right hand on the medial epicondylar area of the patient's femur and the heel of her right hand against the lateral epicondyle of his tibia (*Figure 8.36*).

Method

The method for this technique is identical with that described for lateral movement, with the forearms being parallel, but this time the physiotherapist's left forearm is below her right forearm.

Medial rotation***

When used in the treatment of extremely painful joints this technique can be very effective. Medial rotation of the tibia on the femur as a grade I movement can be produced either by anteroposterior pressure against the anterior surface of the medial tibial condyle or by postero-anterior pressure against the posterior surface of the lateral condyle or by a combination of both. In the case of the first, the starting position and method are the same as described for antero-posterior movement (*see* page 238) except that the thumbs are placed anteriorly on the medial condyle. If the movement is produced by postero-anterior pressure against the lateral condyle the technique is the same as mentioned above for postero-anterior pressure except that the pressure is applied only to the lateral condyle (*see Figure 8.32*, page 240).

Grade IV in flexion is the next most useful technique for medial rotation. It can be performed with the patient supine or prone.

IN FLEXION SUPINE***

Starting position

The physiotherapist stands by the patient's right hip, facing his feet, flexes his right hip and knee to a right angle and holds the knee between

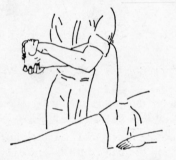

Figure 8.37. – Tibiofemoral medial rotation supine

her left arm and her side. With her left hand pronated she holds his forefoot from the lateral side and with her right hand holds posteriorly and medially around his heel (*Figure 8.37*).

Method

The medial rotation movement is produced by a pulling action of both hands while she stabilizes his knee against her body. Large amplitude movements involving 30 degrees of movement can easily be performed. Small oscillatory grade IV stretching movements can also be performed easily in this position.

It should be appreciated that the technique also includes foot and ankle movement while producing rotation of the knee.

IN FLEXION PRONE***

Starting position

The patient lies prone near the edge of the couch and the physiotherapist stands by his right thigh, facing his feet. She flexes his knee to a right angle and places the heel of her right hand against the medial

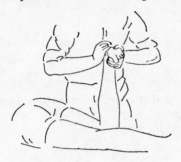

Figure 8.38. – Tibiofemoral medial rotation prone

surface of his heel and her fingers over the sole of his heel with the tips reaching the lateral surface. With her left hand she grasps the dorsum of his forefoot with the heel of her hand against the lateral border and her thumb over the sole. If strong movements are to be used she crouches over his foot to direct her forearms opposite each other (*Figure 8.38*).

Method

Small or large amplitudes can be produced by a pulling and pushing action of both hands in opposite directions. It is essential to prevent the forefoot inverting when pressure is applied to its lateral surface by the left hand.

As with the preceding technique, movement takes place in the foot and ankle as well as the knee. This does not make it any less effective in producing knee rotation. However, if the foot or ankle is painful the knee rotation may need to be produced by grasping the malleoli.

Lateral rotation**

This movement need not be described because its technique and application are similar to medial rotation. For grade I movements postero-anterior and anteroposterior pressures can be used against the appropriate surfaces of the tibia, and the stronger movements in knee flexion can be performed with the patient supine or prone as described above for medial rotation.

Longitudinal movement caudad***

This movement is used in treatment in two main ways. One method is used for very painful knees when grade I movements are given and the other method is used in conjunction with other knee movements. When combined with other movements, it may be included either to make the technique more comfortable or to provide maximum gapping of the joint surfaces. Gapping is often used in conjunction with abduction, extension and rotation.

Starting position

The patient lies near the right-hand edge of the couch with his knee supported in a few degrees of flexion by a pillow. The physiotherapist,

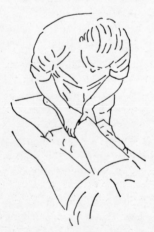

*Figure 8.39. – Tibiofemoral longitudinal
movement caudad*

standing by his right foot, facing his knee, grasps around the head of his tibia with both hands so that her thumbs overlap to reach the opposite side of the tibial tubercle. Her fingers reach around the medial and lateral borders of the tibia to the posterior surface (*Figure 8.39*).

Method

Tiny amplitude oscillations are produced by pulling lightly on the head of the tibia in line with the shaft of the femur.

Longitudinal movement cephalad**

Occasionally compression of the joint surfaces may be useful when included with other accessory movements in the treatment of a painful joint. To effect improvement in such a joint, treatment may require a technique which reduces the pain. This may require including compression of the joint surfaces while applying other movement techniques.

The starting position is the same as that described for longitudinal movement but the compression is provided by the physiotherapist's hands against the head of the tibia moving it towards the head of the femur with an oscillatory movement.

TREATMENT

Although longitudinal movement cephalad and caudad and compression are not frequently used as solo techniques in treatment they may be used in conjunction with abduction/adduction, rotation or flexion/extension movements. An example of this, described by Cyriax[1], is the combination of longitudinal movement caudad and rotation used in attempts to reduce displaced menisci. The techniques which can be used in the treatment of knee conditions are varied. They extend from the gentlest mobilizations using grade I antero-posterior movements for extremely painful knees to the stronger grade IV+ stretching type mobilizations or to the techniques referred to above for the reduction of internal derangements.

[1] Cyriax, J. (1975) *Textbook of Orthopaedic Medicine*, Vol. II. 6th edition. London; Baillière

Treatment by knee extension

Knee conditions referred for physiotherapy frequently present with a lack of active full-range extension and even if the range passively is full it is usually painful with overpressure. The degree of pain felt on extension will frequently be found to be less than the degree of pain which can be produced (with less overpressure) when abduction is combined with the extension. The same is true of flexion compared with flexion/adduction and flexion/abduction. Extension is commonly more positive than flexion. As some people normally experience pain if overpressure is applied to passive knee extension it is proper to compare the disordered knee with the normal knee. It is not commonly realized how much overpressure the normal knee can accept and therefore physiotherapists may frequently miss an abnormality of knee movements. It is therefore necessary to emphasize that one should be prepared to carry out fairly vigorous knee extension tests provided these are done under the right circumstances and are progressed from exploratory gentle extension movements through stages of increasing pressure. Provided the movement is a slow controlled movement the patient will have both the time and the muscular ability to prevent a too strong pressure being applied. In fact it is quite extraordinary how strong the knee flexors are even when the knee is hyperextended.

By reference to any text of anatomy or biomechanics it is understood and accepted that as the knee is actively extended, the tibia, with its concave surface, slides forwards on the convex condyles of the femur. It would seem from this that if passive stretching is being applied to improve the range of extension the physiotherapist should place one hand on the anterior distal surface of the femur pushing it towards the floor while her other hand lifts under the patient's heel. This would permit the anterior surface of the proximal end of the tibia to move anteriorly on the tibial condyles. In the clinical situation however, as compared with the academic situation, better improvement in the range of knee extension will be obtained if the physiotherapist places her hand not on the femur but on the tubercle of the tibia. It is also interesting and important to note that if the technique is performed with one hand on the tibia rather than the femur the stretching technique will be more painful and therefore a more 'comparable sign'. As this pain is always a more 'comparable joint sign', it is therefore an important guide to the amount of overpressure which should be given in the treatment and as a measure for progress.

Another interesting aspect to the use of knee extension as a treatment technique is that if the patient has pain and slight restriction on knee extension and has also some limitation of knee flexion and an active extension 'lag' then passive extension treatment techniques consistently restore the active extension to full range without giving any exercises and also flexion usually recovers at the same time. To gain this improvement in extension lag and knee flexion it is a necessary corollary that by using the knee extension as the treatment technique (with or without adduction or abduction) the passive knee extension will increase in range and the pain will disappear.

Treatment of knee pain

When a patient has a very painful knee which is made worse with walking, or has increased pain with the first few steps following rest, the treatment techniques are directed towards treating pain. The accessory movements which can be used include longitudinal movement cephalad and caudad, postero-anterior and anteroposterior movements, and medial and lateral transverse movements. These would be performed with the knee supported in some degree of flexion and the physiotherapist would use her thumbs to make small amplitude oscillatory movements short of causing any pain or discomfort. Although it is not an accessory movement the technique which is most successful in the treatment of this kind of disorder is rotation. The most comfortable method for this technique would be to place an easily moulded pillow under the supine patient's knee. The physiotherapist would then hold over the top of the patient's knee so that she can feel the medial and lateral coronary ligament with her middle finger and thumb, her palm being over the patella, while with her other hand she comfortably grasps around the medial and lateral malleoli. Starting from a neutral mid position for rotation she would gently and slowly rotate the tibia through approximately 5 degrees of medial rotation and then rotate laterally from that position to 5 degrees of lateral rotation from the mid position. This rotary oscillation would be continued from side to side smoothly and slowly while at the same time feeling the proximal end of the tibia rotating back and forth under her finger and thumb. While performing the movement she should ask the patient whether he feels any sign of discomfort, rubbing or movement. Ideally, the patient should feel nothing but if the physiotherapist has any doubts about what he might be feeling, she should perform exactly the same technique on the other knee and ask him whether the feeling in both knees with the same amplitude of movement is the same. For initial treatment to be successful there should be no difference in the feeling within both knees. If this can be achieved the technique should be performed on the painful knee for no longer than one minute. The patient should be warned of the possibility of exacerbation following the first treatment. At the next treatment session, if there has been any exacerbation, the amplitude should be made smaller and distraction should be added to the technique. If there has been no exacerbation then the amplitude can be increased and perhaps even taken into a small degree of discomfort. From this point on the treatment can be progressed along the same lines as outlined in Chapter 5.

Knee flexion

When, due to trauma, knee flexion is markedly limited though not very painful, and knee extension is full range and painless with strong overpressure, then the principles of treatment are applied as outlined in Chapter 5. That is, knee flexion is the technique used as a sustained stretching small amplitude movement at the limit of the range interspersed with grade IV accessory movements at the limit of the flexion range.

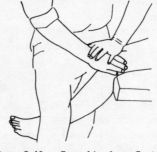

Figure 8.40. – Stretching knee flexion

Another technique which can usefully be used is shown in *Figure 8.40*. The technique involves holding the patient's knee at the limit of flexion, and even stretched further, by the physiotherapist's legs. This leaves her two hands free to stabilize the patella with one hand while applying very strong stretching oscillatory movements against the superior border of the patella, attempting to move it distally as strongly as possible.

PATELLOFEMORAL JOINT

The four main movements of the patella are longitudinal movement cephalad and caudad, and transverse movement medially and laterally. In practice it may be necessary to combine them in pairs to produce diagonal movements cephalad or caudad to elicit pain. When these movements are full range and painless, compression of the patella against the femur should be added to the test movements to elicit the pain.

Whereas transverse movements medially or laterally are best tested or performed in treatment by thumb pressures against the external medial border of the patella, longitudinal movements are more comfortably performed by hand pressures.

Table 8.3
Patellofemoral Joint: Objective Examination

[The knee movements should also be examined as part of the examination of the P/F joint]

Observation

Active movements
>Active quick tests (standing knee F and E; as applicable, squat)
>*Routinely*
>>Gait, stairs
>>Lumbar spine
>>Sitting knee E from F
>>Muscle power through range (weak, pain inhibited, painful arc)
>>Extension lag

Static tests

Other joints in 'plan'

Passive movements
Physiological movements
>*Routinely*
>>Knee F, E, ⟳ , ⟲ in F and E
Accessory movements
>*Routinely*
>>1. Lift and compress
>>2. ⟶ , ⟵ (and vary angles)
>>3. ⟶ ceph and caud each (add med and lat inclinations)
>>Note range, pain, resistance, spasm and behaviour
>*As applicable*
>>1. Above movements with compression
>>2. ⟶ , ceph, caud and angled with knee in different angles of flexion

Palpation

Check case records etc.

HIGHLIGHT MAIN FINDINGS WITH ASTERISKS

After treatment

EXAMINATION

QUICK TESTS

A useful functional test for assessing range and pain is to ask the patient to squat. When the patient reaches the limit of his range the physiotherapist immediately estimates the angle of knee flexion then asks the patient to stand upright again. It should be determined whether any pain or discomfort was felt during the test squatting and why the patient was unable to go further. Perhaps he felt his knees were too weak to allow him to bend further or it may have been due to pain or stiffness.

The behaviour of pain or stiffness will determine the kind of examination and treatment used. For example, if the patient was able to squat fully without any discomfort then the special tests used in examination may need to be vigorous. However, if he was able only to squat through say 40 degrees of knee flexion, with increasing pain eventually limiting the squat, then gentle passive patellofemoral movements should be used in examination and treatment.

Following the quick test of squatting, it is very interesting to compare the available range of non-weight-bearing knee flexion while the patient is in the supine position. Often there is quite a marked difference.

Another facet of patellofemoral movement worthy of including in examination is to ask the patient to extend his knee into the fully hyperextended position while sitting on a table or couch with his thighs supported and his lower legs pendant. Frequently an arc of pain presents midway through the range. If the movement is painless, however, it is worth repeating the knee extension against the physiotherapist's resistance applied at the distal end of the tibia.

SPECIAL TESTS

The purpose of special tests is to move the patella through a full amplitude of movement, as in any radius of a circle, while applying a compressive force against the anterior surface of the patella, thereby rubbing the posterior surface of the patella against the tibia.

TECHNIQUES

Compression**

Starting position

The patient lies supine with a pillow under his knee. The physiotherapist places one hand under the posterior surface of the femur distally, and then places the heel of her other hand over the patella. The centre of the patella should fit between the physiotherapist's thenar and hypothenar eminences and her forearm should be directed vertically through the patient's knee (*Figure 8.41*).

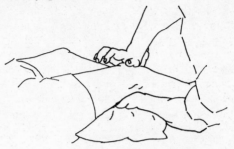

Figure 8.41. – Patellofemoral compression

Method

The technique is one of gently squeezing the patella against the femur. Pressure should be applied gently and slowly against the patella, the patient being asked to report any feeling of discomfort or pain as the pressure is applied.

If no discomfort is felt, maximum pressure can be applied against the patella and a strong small amplitude grade IV+ movement produced.

When this technique is painless or only minimally painful, then a technique can be used where the patella is hit sharply by the heel of the physiotherapist's hand so as to knock the patella sharply against the femur. The first session should be very short (not exceeding 20 seconds) and an assessment made on the following day to guide whether stronger techniques can be used or whether, because an exacerbation has been caused, gentler techniques are indicated.

Transverse movements medially***

Starting position

The physiotherapist stands by the patient's right knee and places the pads of her thumbs, pointing towards each other, against the lateral border of the patella. The fingers of her left and right hands point medially to rest across the distal end of the femur and proximal end of

the tibia respectively. Her thumbs are hyperextended at the interphalangeal joints to bring as much of the pad as possible into contact
with the lateral border of the patella (*Figure 8.42*).

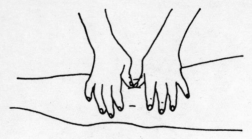

*Figure 8.42. – Patellofemoral articulation;
transverse movement medially*

Method

Oscillatory movements are imparted to the patella through the physiotherapist's thumbs by her arms. If grade I movements are required,
small amplitude oscillations of less than a quarter of an inch from the
normal resting position of the patella are performed. For other grades
of movement the patella is displaced more medially, reaching the limit
of its excursion for grade III and IV movements.

Transverse movements laterally***

These movements are merely the reverse of the above and do not
require description.

Longitudinal movement caudad***

Starting position

The physiotherapist stands by the patient's right knee and places the
heel of her left hand near the pisiform bone, against the superior margin
of the patella. With her left wrist extended she directs her forearm
distally. She places her right hand pointing proximally over the patella
with her fingers and thumb passing either side of the heel of her left
hand. Her right hand serves three purposes: it provides stability for the

left hand, it guides the patella during movement and it can be used to apply compression to the patella when desired (*Figure 8.43*). If stronger techniques are used the physiotherapist should face the patient's feet.

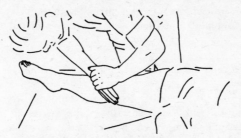

Figure 8.43. – Patellofemoral articulation;
longitudinal movement caudad

Method

The depression movement of the patella is produced by the heel of the physiotherapist's left hand while the direction of the movement is guided by her right hand. Her two hands and his patella move as a single unit. If compression is required during the movement, the patella is firmly pressed against the femur by the physiotherapist's right hand.

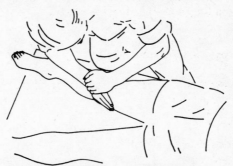

Figure 8.44. – Patellofemoral articulation;
longitudinal movement combined with a
medial inclination and compression

If the movement signs indicate that the movement described above should be combined with a medial inclination, she moves her point of contact against the superior border of the patella slightly laterally and alters the direction of her arms to lie in the direction of the diagonal movement (*Figure 8.44*).

Distraction**

Distraction is the term used to indicate that the patella is lifted away from the femur so that there is no contact between them. This is a very gentle procedure and movements longitudinally, medially and laterally, can be performed very gently in the distracted position.

Starting position

The patient lies supine with his knee extended. The physiotherapist places both thumbs in the space between the patella and femur medially (or laterally). She then places her index fingers in the space on the opposite side. A combination of two acts is necessary to progress to the next stage of the starting position. She should gently squeeze her fingers and thumbs together to reach under the patella, at the same time extending and radially deviating both wrists so that her fingers and thumbs lift against the under surface of the patella (*Figure 8.45a* and *b*).

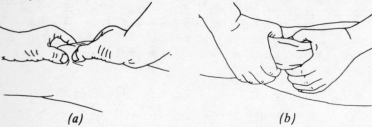

(a)   (b)

Figure 8.45. – Patellofemoral distraction

Method

The technique is a very gentle slow oscillatory movement involving raising and lowering the patella. The patella should not be lowered to the extent where it comes into full contact with the femur. While performing the technique by repeated oscillations, care should be taken to avoid discomfort under the patella.

The above technique can be progressed by the physiotherapist, after having lifted the patella, by moving it medially, laterally, cephalad or caudad. As a modification it is also useful to produce diagonal movements as shown with the other techniques in this chapter.

TREATMENT

The treatment of patellofemoral disorders calls for a high degree of skill and considerable delicacy. When patellofemoral movement is painful the initial session or sessions need to be carried out extremely gently. It is far better to perform movements too gently and for too short a time than to find out at the following session that they had been performed excessively even to the smallest degree. If the physiotherapist has any doubt as to how gently she should begin, then oscillatory distraction should be her first choice. Once the effect of this has been assessed she can then progress in small steps without causing any exacerbation.

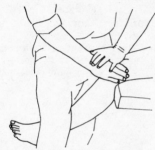

Figure 8.46. – Strong patellofemoral movement

On the other hand, there are times when maximum amplitude movements should be performed in one or more directions, at the same time maintaining a strong compressive force on the patella.

If it is found on examination that the patient is able to squat fully without pain and all examination tests have revealed only minimal signs, it may be necessary to move the patella quite forcibly while the tibiofemoral joint is flexed 40 degrees or more and compression is applied both by the physiotherapist's hand and by resisting the patient's knee extension. This would be done with the patient in the sitting position (*Figure 8.46*).

SUPERIOR TIBIOFIBULAR JOINT

The superior tibiofibular joint is frequently forgotten when seeking the source of lateral leg and knee pain. Although not a frequent cause of pain, it is sufficiently common to warrant inclusion in routine examination. The two movements which can be tested and used in treatment are postero-anterior movement and anteroposterior movement. When these two movements are found to be painless they should be tested while the joint is compressed.

There are no quick tests for the superior tibiofibular joint. However, the two quick tests referred to above, that is, vigorous postero-anterior movement and anteroposterior movement, both performed with very strong compression, are quite effective.

Table 8.4 lists the examination for the superior tibiofibular joint.

Table 8.4
Superior Tibiofibular Joint: Objective Examination

[The knee movements should also be examined as part of the examination for the superior tibiofibular (T/F) joint. Ankle joint movements should also be checked as the superior tibiofibular joint moves with full range ankle movements]

Observation

Active movements

Static tests

Other structures in 'plan'
   Entrapment neuropathy

Passive movements
Accessory movements
   Routinely

   ↕ , ↕ , ↔ ceph and caud (by ankle inversion and eversion)
   Note range, pain, resistance, spasm and behaviour

   As applicable
   1. Repeat above, adding compression
   2. Repeat ↕ , ↕ , ↔ ceph and caud by lying on side using hand for
      1V+ with compression

Palpation
   Entrapment neuropathy

Check case records etc.

HIGHLIGHT MAIN FINDINGS WITH ASTERISKS

After treatment

Anteroposterior movement***

Starting position

The patient lies with his right hip and knee flexed and his foot resting on the couch. The physiotherapist sits on his foot to stabilize it and places her thumbs against the anterior border of the head of the fibula. Both thumbs point posteriorly with the tips in contact with the head of the fibula (*Figure 8.47a*).

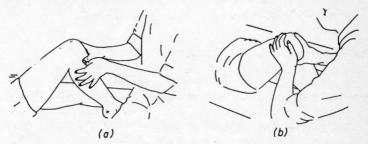

(a)   *(b)*

Figure 8.47. – Superior tibiofibular (a) anteroposterior movement; (b) anteroposterior movement with compression

Method

Anteroposterior pressures are exerted against the head of the fibula through stable thumbs. It is extremely difficult to differentiate between different grades of movement but they can be varied by altering the strength of the pressures.

If the addition of compression is necessary, the heel of the left hand is placed over the head of the fibula laterally while the fingers lie over the knee. The right thumb maintains its contact against the anterior margin of the fibula. The left forearm is directed so that it can apply a medially directed pressure against the head of the fibula as well as assisting the right thumb in its anteroposterior pressure (*Figure 8.47b*).

Postero-anterior movement***

For examination purposes postero-anterior movement can be tested with the patient supine with his knee and hip flexed as described above. A pulling pressure is then applied behind the head of the fibula. However, when this movement is used for treatment the patient should lie prone.

Starting position

The patient lies prone near the right-hand edge of the couch. The physiotherapist, standing alongside the patient's foot, places her left knee on the couch and supports his right lower leg across her thigh. This position supports the patient's knee in approximately 30 degrees of flexion. She then places the pads of her thumbs against the posterior border of the head of his fibula, with the fingers of her left hand spreading medially across his upper calf and those of her right hand reaching anteriorly around the fibula (*Figure 8.48a*).

Method

Postero-anterior mobilizing is performed by pressure from the physiotherapist's arms acting through her thumbs against the head of the fibula. It is essential that she should not produce movement with the muscles of her thumbs as this immediately becomes uncomfortable to the patient.

The movement can be performed under compression by changing the position of the physiotherapist's right hand so that the heel of the hand is placed against the lateral surface of the head of the fibula (*Figure 8.48b*).

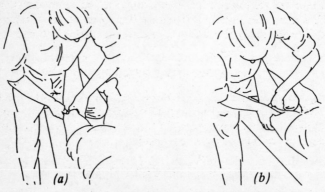

*Figure 8.48. – Superior tibiofibular (a) postero-anterior movement;
(b) postero-anterior movement with compression*

Longitudinal movement cephalad and caudad

Starting position

The patient lies prone with his knee flexed to a right angle. The physiotherapist holds the patient's foot in her hands and produces caudad longitudinal movement by strongly inverting the patient's heel. A cephalad longitudinal movement is produced by the physiotherapist everting the patient's heel. This movement can readily be felt in the normal subject by palpating the head of the fibula with one hand while inverting and everting the patient's heel with the other hand.

TREATMENT

Little comment need be made on treatment of superior tibiofibular joint problems. It is not very easy to determine whether the superior tibiofibular joint is responsible for a patient's symptoms and frequently this can only be ascertained by performing strong techniques with strong compression and comparing these on the faulty leg with symptoms felt when repeated on the good leg. When a comparable sign is found this movement should be used in treatment. Initially it should be performed firmly but not vigorously. If the test signs are obvious then the postero-anterior or anteroposterior movements should be performed without compression. It is quite common, however, for the techniques to be performed with strong compression. When this is necessary the movements should be reasonably vigorous and may need to be repeated for four groups, each lasting approximately one minute.

When the inferior tibiofibular joint is responsible for symptoms, it responds very readily and rapidly to passive mobilizing techniques.

COMPOSITE KNEE JOINT

Having discussed in detail the examination and treatment techniques for the tibiofemoral joint, the patellofemoral joint and the superior tibiofibular joint, it may be helpful to summarize the examination for the three joints (Table 8.5 on next page).

INFERIOR TIBIOFIBULAR JOINT

The inferior tibiofibular joint is more frequently the cause of symptoms than the superior tibiofibular joint and should be routinely examined when ankle pain is present.

The movements described relate to movement of the fibula on the larger more stable tibia. The movements are anteroposterior and postero-anterior movement of the fibula on the tibia which, during examination, may require testing while the joint surfaces are compressed. Strong rotation of the talus (produced via the foot) also produces movement at the tibiofibular joint as does compressing the talus into the mortice.

Table 8.5
Composite Knee Joint: Objective Examination

Observation

Active quick tests
　　　　Gait: forwards, backwards, on heels (esp. backwards), on toes
　　　　Squat: on toes, on feet flat, bounce
　　　　Height of step possible
　　　　On all fours sit towards heels
　　　　Sit, resist available extension
　　　　Supine, quads lag

Static tests
　　　　Of quads in different ranges of F/E

Other joints in 'plan'

Passive movements
　　　Tibiofemoral joint
　　　　1.　E, E/Ab, E/Ad, Ab, Ad, F, F/Ab, F/Ad
　　　　2.　↕ and ↕ , ↦ and ↤ in 90 degrees knee flexion
　　　　3.　↻ ↺ in knee F and E
　　　Patellofemoral joint
　　　　1.　↦ ↤ in knee F and E
　　　　2.　↠ ceph, caud, ↘ ↗ ↖ ↗ with and without compression
　　　　3.　In sitting (knee F 90 degrees) ↠ ceph, caud, ↘ ↗ ↖ ↗ with and
　　　　　　without compression
　　　Superior tibiofibular joint
　　　　1.　↕ ↕ with and without compression
　　　　2.　↠ ceph and caud (by ankle Inv and Ev) with and without compression

Palpation

Check case records etc.

HIGHLIGHT MAIN FINDINGS WITH ASTERISKS

After treatment

Longitudinal movement can be produced by inverting and everting the
heel (*see* page 260). It must also be remembered that the 'close-packed'
position which spreads the inferior tibiofibular joint is produced by
anteroposterior movement of the talus (*see Figure 8.63*, page 281) as
well as dorsiflexion. The full examination is listed in Table 8.6.

Table 8.6
Inferior Tibiofibular Joint: Objective Examination

[Movements of the ankle joint should also be examined as part of the examination for the inferior T/F joint]

Observation

Active movements
    Active quick tests
    Routinely
    Gait, heel and toe walking forwards and backwards, hopping (esp. heel), squatting
    DF, PF; Inv and Ev
    Note range and pain

Static tests

Other structures in 'plan'
    Full active resisted movements through range for 'sheaths'
    Joint restriction c.f. muscle/tendon restriction

Passive movements
Physiological movements
    Routinely
    Ankle DF, PF, Inv, Ev
    Note range, pain, resistance, spasm and behaviour
    As applicable
    The injuring movement
Accessory movements
Routinely
    1. Ankle ↨ , ↿ , ↻ , ↺ , ↔ ceph and caud, Inv, Ev
    2. T/F
        (a) ↨ , ↿ , with and without compression
        (b) ↔ ceph and caud (by using ankle Inv and Ev) with and without compression

    Note range, pain, resistance, spasm and behaviour

As applicable
    ↓ and ↿ with compression

Palpation
    Palpate tendon sheaths

Check case records etc.

HIGHLIGHT MAIN FINDINGS WITH ASTERISKS

After treatment

EXAMINATION

QUICK TESTS

There are two main quick tests though there are many other movements the patient can be asked to do which will guide the kind of examination.

The first quick test is to ask the patient to squat while keeping his heels on the floor. In this position the mortice joint is jammed into the close-packed position, thus spreading the inferior tibiofibular joint apart, while the patient's bodyweight is being taken through this area.

The second quick test is to ask the patient to walk on his heels. If he can do this, he should attempt hopping on the heel of the painful foot.

SPECIAL TESTS

There are no specific special tests for this joint other than the movements described in the following text.

TECHNIQUES

Postero-anterior movement***

Starting position

The patient lies prone with his right knee flexed to a right angle. The physiotherapist stands by his right knee, facing his left thigh, and places the heel of her pronated right hand against the posterior border of the lateral malleolus and the heel of her left hand against the anterior border of the medial malleolus. The fingers of her right hand are directed forward towards his toes and the fingers of her left hand towards his heel. Both forearms are directed opposite each other and parallel to the central axis of the patient's trunk (*Figure 8.49a*).

Method

Oscillatory mobilizations, which are only possible in small amplitude, are produced by the physiotherapist's arms exerting alternating pressure and relaxation against the malleoli.

WITH COMPRESSION***

Compression can be applied during this movement by the physiotherapist adjusting her position so that she faces his left hip and directs her forearms diagonally through the ankle (*Figure 8.49b*).

GRADES I AND II** If extremely gentle movements are required, she should support the distal end of the patient's tibia in her left hand as described above with the heel of her hand against the anterior surface, while the pad of her right thumb is placed behind the lateral malleolus with her fingers spreading medially for stability (*Figure 8.49c*). The mobilization is then produced by the right arm acting through the thumb.

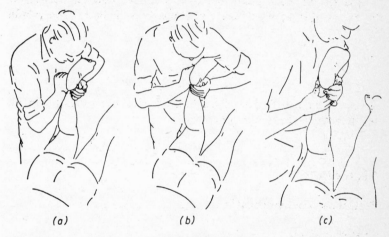

(a)   *(b)*   *(c)*

Figure 8.49. – Inferior tibiofibular (a) postero-anterior movement; (b) postero-anterior movement with compression; (c) grades I and II postero-anterior movement with thumb

ALTERNATIVE METHOD

An alternative method of producing postero-anterior movement which some physiotherapists may find easier to perform is now described. It is certainly a much easier position in which to use grades IV and IV+ stretching techniques and one in which it is easy to add the compression component.

Starting position

The patient lies on his left side and flexes his hip and knee to a right angle so that the medial surface of his lower leg and foot are lying flat on the table. The physiotherapist stands behind the patient's leg and uses two hands to apply pressure against the posterior border of the lateral malleolus. Her hands work together as a single unit, performing a very localized technique in which only her pisiform contacts the lateral malleolus posteriorly (*Figure 8.50*).

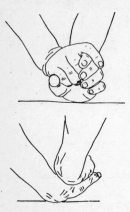

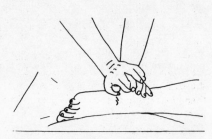

Figure 8.50. – *Inferior tibiofibular postero-anterior movement, alternative method*

Method

The physiotherapist uses her body to transmit the movement to the fibula while her elbows act as springs.

Anteroposterior movement**

Starting position

The patient lies prone with his knee flexed to a right angle. The physiotherapist stands by his knee, facing his left lower leg, and places the heel of her fully pronated left hand against the anterior surface of the lateral malleolus with her fingers spreading posteriorly around his ankle. She places the heel of her supinated right hand against the posterior surface of the medial malleolus with her fingers spreading anteriorly around the ankle. Her forearms are directed opposite each other parallel to the central axis of the trunk (*Figure 8.51a*).

Method

The small amplitude oscillatory mobilization is produced by the physiotherapist's forearms applying equal and opposite pressures through her hands. She will have more control of the movement if she crouches over her hands.

Variation for anteroposterior and postero-anterior movements

When firm techniques are required the patient is asked to lie on his side with his hip and knee comfortably flexed so as to allow the medial surface of his leg to rest on the couch. The physiotherapist stands behind the patient's leg for postero-anterior movements, and in front of his leg for anteroposterior movements. She places the heel of one hand (the emphasis of the contact being through the pisiform) against the lateral malleolus.

The physiotherapist then uses her bodyweight to move the lateral malleolus in relation to the tibia. By varying the direction of her arms she can produce a postero-anterior or anteroposterior movement and then by raising her arms she can add varying amounts of compression to the movement.

In this position she is also able to direct her pressure on the lateral malleolus towards the patient's head or towards his feet so that a component of longitudinal movement, either cephalad or caudad, can also be incorporated.

The technique is the same as that described for the inferior tibio-fibular joint in the side-lying position (*see* page 266, *Figure 8.50*).

WITH COMPRESSION***

To apply compression during anteroposterior movement, she alters her position to face his left foot and directs her forearms diagonally across the central axis of the trunk while still maintaining them in the coronal plane (*Figure 8.51b*).

GRADE II** If extremely gentle movements are required, the physio-therapist should support the distal end of the patient's tibia in her right hand as described above while placing the pad of her left thumb against the anterior border of the lateral malleolus. Her fingers provide stability by their position on the front of the leg. The mobilization is produced by her left arm acting through the thumb (*Figure 8.51c*).

An alternative position for producing this anteroposterior movement may be found easier to perform by some physiotherapists.

Starting position

The patient lies on his left side with his hip and knee flexed so that the medial surface of his lower leg and foot rest evenly on the table.

The physiotherapist stands in front of the patient's foot and places her pisiform against the anterior border of the lateral malleolus (*Figure 8.51d*).

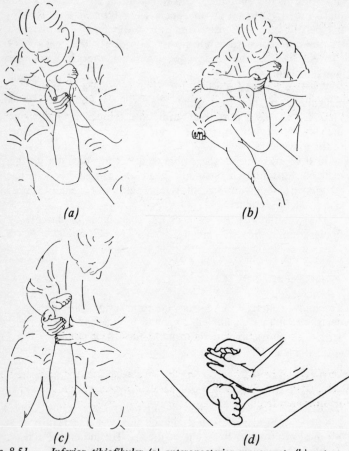

(a)   *(b)*

(c)   *(d)*

Figure 8.51. – Inferior tibiofibular (a) anteroposterior movement; (b) antero-posterior movement with compression; (c) grade II movement with thumbs; (d) grade IV movement with compression

Method

The physiotherapist produces an oscillatory movement of the fibula on the tibia by rocking her body so that her trunk produces movement of her hands against the malleolus. The movement is produced by body movement and not by arm movement.

The physiotherapist can alter the direction of her arm in relation to the malleolus so that the technique is a purely anteroposterior one or she may alter it to include compression.

Compression**

Starting position

The patient lies prone with his knee flexed to a right ankle. The physiotherapist stands beyond his knee, facing his left hip. She bends slightly at the waist to position her left shoulder over his foot, placing the heel

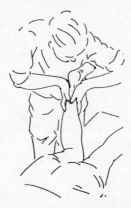

Figure 8.52. – Inferior tibiofibular compression

of her left and right hands over the medial and lateral malleoli respectively, with the fingers of both hands directed towards his knee. Her forearms are directed opposite each other (*Figure 8.52*).

Method

There is very little movement in this direction but a patient with symptoms arising from this joint is well aware of pain during movement. Compression is produced through the operator's forearms by alternating pressures against the malleoli. During treatment it may be necessary for the physiotherapist to alter the direction of her forearms slightly to permit slight anteroposterior or postero-anterior movement of the fibula in relation to the tibia.

Alternative method

The same movement can be performed with the patient lying on his side. The physiotherapist places one hand under the lateral malleolus, cupping it in her palm near the heel of her hand. With her other hand she presses through the medial malleolus, placing the thenar eminence near the heel of her hand against it (*Figure 8.53*).

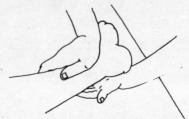

Figure 8.53. – Inferior tibiofibular compression, alternative method

Inferior tibiofibular movement during ankle rotation

When the talus is rotated strongly in the mortise it spreads the inferior tibiofibular joint. Also, during medial rotation, the fibula is pulled anteriorly in relation to the tibia and during lateral rotation it moves posteriorly. The rotation can be produced by the physiotherapist

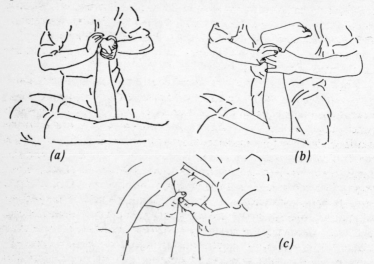

Figure 8.54. – Inferior tibiofibular movement during ankle rotation. (a) Medial rotation using foot leverage; (b) medial talocrural rotation; (c) lateral talocrural rotation

using the patient's heel and foot as a lever (*Figure 8.54a*) and the patient's report of the site of pain will indicate whether the pain is arising from the intertarsal joints, the ankle joint or the inferior tibiofibular joint.

The movement can also be produced by holding the talus between the index finger and thumb of both hands so that the talus can be rotated in the mortise (*Figure 8.54b* and *c*). If pain is reproduced with this movement it is still difficult to discern whether the pain is arising from the ankle joint or the inferior tibiofibular joint.

Heel tap

This technique should be used as an examination procedure routinely when the inferior tibiofibular joint is thought to be contributing to a patient's ankle pain. It consists of hitting the sole of the patient's heel, driving the talus into the mortise and both jarring and spreading the inferior tibiofibular joint. The technique is described in full on page 285 (*see Figure 8.67*).

TREATMENT

When a patient's foot is subjected to fairly severe trauma the inferior tibiofibular joint is often involved in the strain. This fact is frequently overlooked because the condition of the joints below is more severe and more limiting. However, a faulty inferior tibiofibular joint can prevent normal walking and should not be omitted from the routine examination of the foot and ankle.

When the joint is found to be the source of symptoms the examination technique which reproduces the patient's symptoms, or the examination technique which discloses a loss of range, is the technique which should be used in treatment. A treatment session would involve gentle grade IV− type movements interspersed with grade III− movements if pain is a dominant factor. If the aim of treatment is to increase range, the movement needing to be increased should be stretched as a strong IV+ movement. Following approximately one minute of this strongly performed technique, the joint should be held in this position of stretch, while grade IV+ accessory movements are stretched in each direction. Following the accessory movement stretches, the stretching of the stiff physiological movement should be repeated as a grade IV+ movement. The total stretching treatment will consist of alternating between stretching the physiological movement and stretching the accessory movements while the joint is held at the limit of the physiological range.

ANKLE JOINT

When learning movements and techniques of the foot it is advisable to have an articulated set of bones available (*Figures 8.55* and *8.56*).

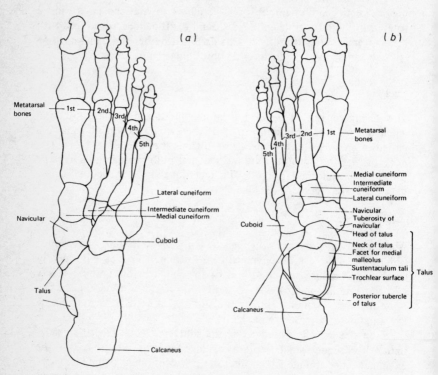

Figure 8.55. – The skeleton of the left foot (a) plantar aspect; (b) dorsal aspect. (Reproduced by courtesy of Gray's Anatomy (1973), pp. 374, 375. 35th Edition. Edinburgh; Churchill Livingstone)

During examination and treatment of the ankle joint, the required movements are more easily performed by using the foot as a lever, thus incorporating intertarsal movement with talocrural movement. However, mobilization techniques are most effective if they are localized to the movement of the faulty joint. During most techniques, movement can be isolated to the hindfoot (that is the calcaneum and talus) but it is sometimes difficult to differentiate completely between subtalar and ankle movement disorders.

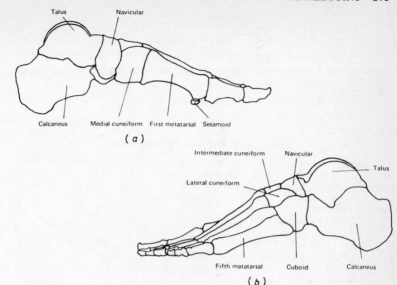

Figure 8.56. – The skeleton of the left foot. (a) medial aspect; (b) lateral aspect. (Reproduced by courtesy of Gray's Anatomy (1973), p. 469. 35th Edition. Edinburgh; Churchill Livingstone)

EXAMINATION

The accessory movements which should be examined at the ankle joint are anteroposterior and postero-anterior movements of the talus, longitudinal movement cephalad and caudad of the talus within the ankle joint and rotation. The physiological movements are inversion (or adduction), eversion (or abduction), dorsiflexion and plantar flexion.

QUICK TESTS

The patient should first be asked to squat, without specific directive. If he squats fully with his heels off the ground then he should be asked to squat again, keeping his heels on the ground as this forces greater dorsiflexion. Squatting having been assessed, the patient should then be asked to walk forwards, away from and then towards the physiotherapist. This should be followed by walking backwards, away from then towards the physiotherapist.

If the above tests reveal no abnormality the patient should be asked to walk on his toes and then on his heels. This should be followed by hopping on the toes of the disordered foot and then hopping on the heel.

SPECIAL TESTS

Careful execution of the accessory movements, noting range and pain, is important in the assessment of ankle disorders. An accessory movement which is frequently forgotten is that of longitudinal movement caudad (*see Figure 8.68*, page 286).

The full examination is listed in Table 8.7.

Table 8.7
Ankle Joint: Objective Examination

[As hind foot intertarsal movements must be examined as part of the examination of the ankle joint it is simpler to describe them together. The inferior T/F joint should also be examined]

Active movements
    Active quick tests
    Routinely
        Gait, heel and toe walking forwards and backwards, heel and toe hopping, squatting (spontaneous then flat heels)
        DF, PF, Inv, Ev
        Note range and pain

Static tests

Other structures in 'plan'
    Full active resisted movements through range for 'sheaths'
    Joint restriction c.f. muscle/tendon restriction

Passive movements
Physiological movements
    Routinely
        DF, PF, Inv, Ev
    As applicable
        DF and PF differentiating
        Inv and Ev differentiating
Accessory movements
    Routinely
        ⊃ , ⊂ , ↿ , ⇂ , ↔ ceph and caud, with and without compression
        ↔ ↔ subtaloid varying inclinations, ⇂ , ↿
        Note range, pain, resistance, spasm and behaviour
    As applicable
        Differentiating ⊃ , ⊂ , ↿ , ⇂ , ↔ ceph and caud

Palpation
    Include tendon sheaths

Check case records etc.

HIGHLIGHT MAIN FINDINGS WITH ASTERISKS

After treatment

TECHNIQUES

Plantar flexion***

Starting position

The patient lies prone with his knee flexed to a right angle while the physiotherapist, standing by his knee, holds his calcaneum posteriorly in her right hand and anteriorly over the neck of the talus in her left hand. She places her left knee on the couch to support his right shin, a position which greatly assists relaxation. With her right hand she holds his calcaneum with her thumb around the lateral surface, her medial three fingers around the medial surface and her index finger, especially the palmar surface of the metacarpophalangeal joint, firmly contracting the sole. She places the web of the first interosseous space of her left hand over the neck of the talus adjacent to his ankle so that her thumb rests against the lateral side of his foot and her fingers against the medial malleolus. Both arms remain near her side as she stands near his foot (*Figure 8.57*).

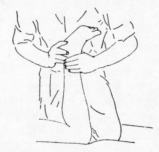

Figure 8.57. — Ankle joint; plantar flexion

Method

Plantar flexion movements of small or large amplitude are easily controlled from this position and can be performed in any part of the range. The movements are performed by her arms.

If movement of the forefoot (that is that part of the foot distal to the navicular bone) is to be included, the physiotherapist places her left hand more distally on the dorsum of the patient's foot. If grade III+ movements of the whole foot are required, the starting position should be altered as follows.

GRADE III+***

Starting position

The patient lies prone with his feet near the end of the couch. The physiotherapist stands by his feet, facing his head, and holds his right foot in both hands. She places her thumbs, pointing proximally, along

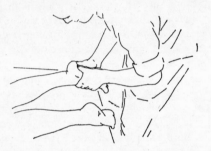

Figure 8.58. – Ankle joint; plantar flexion
grade III+

the medial and lateral borders of the sole of his heel, while her fingers, meeting over the dorsum of his foot, complete the grasp from in front (*Figure 8.58*). The position of the fulcrum provided by the tips of the thumbs may be varied to emphasize the movement to any of the intertarsal or tarsometatarsal joints. To further localize the movement the physiotherapist's fingers would be positioned firmly over the appropriate joint or immediately adjacent distally.

Method

The physiotherapist raises the patient's leg through approximately 20 degrees of knee flexion while partially dorsiflexing his ankle. She then drops his leg through those 20 degrees, at the same time strongly plantar flexing his foot, timing the movement so that the drop of the leg assists the plantar flexion at the limit of range.

When it is necessary to localize the plantar flexion movement to the intertarsal joints, a different grasp of the patient's heel is required. This technique is described with other techniques related to the intertarsal joints (*see* page 299 and *Figure 8.78*).

Dorsiflexion***

Starting position

The patient lies prone with his knee flexed to slightly more than a right angle. The physiotherapist, standing by his right knee with her left knee on the couch to support his shin, holds his calcaneum in her right hand, with her thumb along the lateral surface and her fingers along the medial surface. She uses the web of the first interosseous space of her right hand to grip the calcaneum around its superior surface posteriorly. She places the web of the first interosseous space of her left hand across the plantar surface of his calcaneum distally and laterally, with her thumb passing laterally around his foot and her fingers medially. She directs her right elbow towards the floor and her left towards the ceiling (*Figure 8.59*).

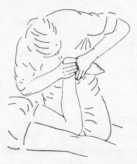

Figure 8.59. – Ankle joint; dorsiflexion

Method

The oscillatory movement is gained by her forearms working in opposite directions producing a dorsiflexion movement about the ankle. This can be performed in any grade although the grasp described above is inadequate for stronger techniques. As the limit of the range is required, flexion of the knee beyond a right angle may be necessary to reduce tension in the gastrocnemius.

GRADES III+ AND IV+*

For stronger techniques the physiotherapist changes her left hand position to use the heel of her hand against the patient's metatarsal heads. The change of position incorporates intertarsal movement with the talocrural movement (*Figure 8.60*).

To localize movement to the intertarsal joints, the physiotherapist adopts a different grasp of the patient's forefoot and heel. This technique is described with other techniques used in the treatment of intertarsal joints (*see* page 286).

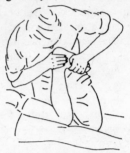

Figure 8.60. – Ankle joint; dorsiflexion, grades III + and IV+

Inversion***

Starting position

The patient lies prone with his knee flexed to a right angle. The physiotherapist, standing by his knee and supporting his shin, grasps his calcaneum with both hands; her thumbs are adjacent to each other

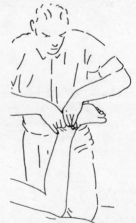

Figure 8.61. – Ankle joint; inversion

pointing proximally on the lateral surface while her fingers hold over the medial surface. The main grasp is between the index and middle fingers medially and the thumb laterally of each hand (*Figure 8.61*). With this grasp of the calcaneum the movement is isolated to the talo-calcanean, the talocrural and the inferior tibiofibular joints.

When the physiotherapist holds around the metatarsals, which is the starting position used for a general inversion-type movement of the whole foot (*see Figure 8.70*, page 291), then supination or rotation takes place at all of the intertarsal and tarsometatarsal joints distal to the talus and calcaneum.

Method

If the technique for large amplitude movements is described first that for smaller amplitudes will not be necessary. To produce a grade III movement, the physiotherapist holds the patient's foot away from her and performs the movement by pulling his leg towards her while at the same time inverting his calcaneum. The movement is performed in such a way that the swinging movement of his leg (which is really a rotary movement of the hip through an arc of approximately 15 degrees) assists the inversion action produced by her wrists.

When inversion is used as a treatment technique the best results are obtained when the movement is localized to the particular faulty joint. However, when a patient has an injured foot and all joints are involved, or when the most comparable joint sign is found with eversion applied through the metatarsals, then the general inversion/adduction/supination movement is the best one to use.

Eversion***

Eversion has an identical starting position with that adopted for inversion. The method also is similar in that eversion of the calcaneum is produced by movement of the physiotherapist's wrists coinciding with swinging the patient's leg away from her. The swinging leg action is lateral rotation of the hip.

Postero-anterior movement**

The postero-anterior direction relates to movement of the foot on the leg.

Starting position

The patient lies with his knee flexed to a right angle. The physiotherapist stands by his knee and supports his right shin against her
left thigh. She holds his calcaneum in her right hand with the heel of
her hand against the posterior surface, her fingers and thumb spreading

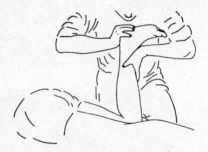

*Figure 8.62. – Ankle joint; postero-
anterior movement*

distally over and around the calcaneum. She places the heel of her
supinated left hand against the anterior surface of the tibia with her
fingers pointing proximally. Her medial two fingers and thumb hold
around the lateral and medial surfaces respectively. She crouches over
his foot to direct her forearms opposite each other parallel to the
central axis of the trunk (*Figure 8.62*).

Method

A large amplitude movement can be produced in this direction but care
must be taken with two things. Firstly, the contact against the tibia
must be made as cushioned as possible by cupping the thenar and
hypothenar eminences, because bone-to-bone contact between the heel
of the hand and the tibia is uncomfortable. Secondly, during the return
part of the postero-anterior movement complete relaxation of the
pressure against the heel is necessary. Useful and effective treatment
movements of grade III+ and IV+ type can be produced at the limit of
the range.

VARIATIONS (MORE LOCALIZED TALOCRURAL)

The technique described above uses the calcaneum as the bone through which the postero-anterior movement is performed. It is therefore obvious that during the technique there will be movement of the subtaloid joint as well as the ankle joint. Usually this is unimportant as the excursion of postero-anterior movement at the subtaloid joint is minimal and nearly always pain free. However, if the movement is being used as an examination technique and when performed it produces pain, then it may be necessary to produce the postero-anterior movement by direct pressure on the talus, thereby avoiding any subtaloid movement.

This localization of the postero-anterior movement is achieved while the patient is still prone with his knee flexed to 90 degrees. The physiotherapist, standing by his hip, places the pads of both thumbs on the talus posterior to the Achilles tendon. With her fingers passing anteriorly around the malleoli to provide counterpressure on the anterior surfaces, she produces the postero-anterior movement with her arms, pushing the talus anteriorly between the malleoli.

Anteroposterior movement**

Starting position

The patient lies prone with his knee flexed to a right angle. The physiotherapist stands by his right knee, supporting his shin, and holds his leg distally from behind in her right hand with her thumb around the fibula and her fingers around the tibia. She positions her left hand with her index finger passing distal to his medial malleolus and her thumb

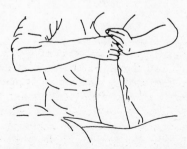

Figure 8.63. — Ankle joint; anteroposterior movement

distal to his lateral malleolus. This places the web of her first inter-osseous space on the neck of the talus. The physiotherapist needs to ensure that the web is tight so that she feels she is grasping the talus around three sides with her index finger, web and thumb. She crouches over his foot and directs her forearms opposite each other, parallel to the central axis of the trunk (*Figure 8.63*).

Method

There is less movement in this direction than there is with postero-anterior movement and it is a movement which is less frequently found to be painful. The movement, in any grade, is produced by an opposite action of both forearms, with the left hand creating most of the movement.

VARIATIONS (MORE LOCALIZED TALOCRURAL)

Starting position

The patient lies supine with his hip and knee flexed and his foot resting on the couch. The physiotherapist stands beyond his foot facing it, and places the pads of her thumbs on the talus immediately between

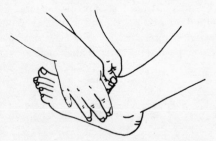

*Figure 8.64. – Ankle joint; localized
anteroposterior movement*

the malleoli. It is more comfortable for the patient if the maximum area of the pads of the thumbs is used rather than the tips of the thumbs (*Figure 8.64*).

Method

Anteroposterior movement of the talus within the mortise is produced by the physiotherapist's trunk and arms and it is transmitted through the talus via the pads of the thumbs. Any concentric muscle action of the thumb flexors will spoil the technique completely. It will make the technique uncomfortable for the patient and the physiotherapist will lose all feel of movement during the technique. When the technique using the thumbs is uncomfortable it may produce discomfort which is difficult to separate from the patient's symptoms felt in the same area.

Medial rotation**

Starting position

The patient lies prone with his right knee flexed to a right angle while the physiotherapist, standing by his right knee, places her left knee on the couch to support his shin. She stabilizes his lower leg anteriorly

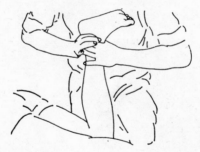

Figure 8.65. – Ankle joint; medial rotation

in her left hand by holding around the medial malleolus with her fingers and placing the pad of her thumb against the anterior surface of the lateral malleolus. With her right hand she endeavours to grasp the talus posteriorly with her index finger passing medially and her thumb laterally. Her thumb and index finger must be adjacent and distal to his malleoli (*Figure 8.65*).

Method

Medial rotation is a very small movement and the difficulty of the grasp results from considerable skin movement. Skin slack must be taken up before movement can be imparted. However, rotation can be produced and it can be an important technique in the mobilization of this joint. The rotation is produced by a screwing action of both arms, her right arm producing the main movement.

Lateral rotation**

Starting position

The patient lies prone with his right knee flexed to a right angle and the physiotherapist stands by his knee holding his foot in her hands. She places her left knee on the couch to support his shin. She stabilizes his lower leg posteriorly with her right hand, hooking her fingers around the medial malleolus to grasp anteriorly while placing the pad of her thumb against the posterior surface of the lateral malleolus. With her left hand she endeavours to grasp the talus anteriorly. She places her index finger immediately adjacent and distal to the medial malleolus and her thumb adjacent and distal to the lateral malleolus (*Figure 8.66*).

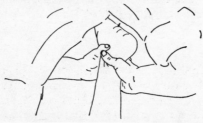

Figure   8.66.   –   *Ankle   joint;   lateral   rotation*

Method

As with medial rotation the movement is small and skin slack must be taken up first. The lateral rotation is produced by the physiotherapist's left hand pivoting the patient's talus around the tibia and fibula which are held stabilized in her right hand.

Longitudinal movement cephalad**

Compression can be a surprisingly useful technique in the treatment of painful ankles when the movement is found to be painful or the patient experiences pain on the 'heel-strike' during walking.

Starting position

The patient lies prone with his right knee flexed to a right angle and the physiotherapist stands by his right knee and supports his shin. She holds his forefoot in her left hand to control the position of dorsiflexion of his ankle (*Figure 8.67*).

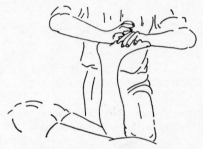

Figure 8.67. – Ankle joint; longitudinal movement cephalad

Method

The physiotherapist imparts the movement by tapping the sole of the heel between the medial and lateral processes of the calcaneum with the pisiform area of the heel of her right hand. When this technique is used in treatment, the strength of the tap and the angle of dorsiflexion are adjusted in order to reproduce the symptoms by the tapping.

Longitudinal movement caudad*

Starting position

The patient lies prone with his knee flexed to a right angle and the physiotherapist stands by his knee. She grasps his talus in her right hand with her thumb laterally, her index finger medially and the web of her first interosseous space stretching across the posterior process. With her left hand she holds the neck of the talus immediately anterior to the ankle joint, with her thumb crossing the lateral surface and her index finger crossing the medial surface. She then gently places her right knee across the posterior surface of his femur distally (*Figure 8.68*).

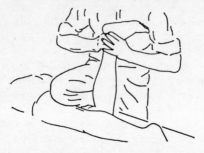

*Figure 8.68. – Ankle joint; longitudinal
movement caudad*

Method

She stabilizes his knee and lifts the talus (and foot) towards the ceiling with both arms. Alternate lifting and releasing is repeated for the period of the mobilization. The technique can be performed gently or strongly in small or large amplitudes anywhere in the range. A patient with symptoms is well aware of movement even when gentle oscillatory movements are performed.

INTERTARSAL MOVEMENT

Movements of the foot involve different movements about different axes in different parts of the foot. The complexity of these movements needs to be understood if the best results from passive movement treatment are to be obtained. All recognized textbooks of anatomy describe the individual movements and most will concur that discrepancies in the description of movements exist. Taking the foot as a unit, inversion and eversion are separately described in this text.

From a clinical point of view, during inversion of the foot, four movements take place.

1.   The heel inverts. (The calcaneum inverts at the subtalar joint, pulling the talus into a range of inversion also. This movement is sometimes referred to as adduction.)

2. Medial rotation. This is a movement of the forefoot on the hind foot at the transverse tarsal joint, the transverse tarsal joint being between the calcaneum and talus proximally and the navicular and cuboid distally. Further medial rotation takes place between the navicular and cuneiform and even at the tarsometatarsal joints. (Medial rotation is often referred to as supination.)

The forefoot, that is, that part of the foot which lies distal to the transverse tarsal joint, is made up largely of the metatarsals. However, the majority of the rotary movement takes place at the transverse tarsal joint when the movement is performed actively. If the movement of inversion is produced passively via the metatarsals then a considerable degree of supination is created between the metatarsals.

3. Adduction. This movement also takes place at the transverse tarsal joint, with the navicular bone sliding medially on the head of the talus. Although this movement is small when the foot is actively inverted, it is possible to produce passively quite a large range of adduction at the transverse tarsal joint and at the navicular cuneiform joints.

4. Plantar flexion. When inversion is performed passively and the maximum range is produced, plantar flexion occurs at three places to allow a greater amount of apparent forefoot movement. The first is at the tarsometatarsal joints and the second part takes place at all of the forefoot joints thus producing a maximum medial facing of the sole of the foot. When the ankle is plantar flexed a greater range of talocrural movement is possible and it is here where a third part of plantar flexion takes place.

During eversion the reverse takes place and the total range of movement is much less.

EXAMINATION

During examination by passive movement all of the above movements can be performed. When any of them produce pain it becomes necessary to examine the movements, both physiological and accessory, which can take place at each metatarsal joint. These tests can be carried out as described in the text which follows and particular emphasis should be placed upon movements produced by thumb pressure on individual bones and by the gliding movements created by holding adjacent bones in each hand and forcing them to glide past each other in opposite directions.

QUICK TESTS

The patient should be asked to squat fully, without being given any other directive. He will squat spontaneously and any abnormality of rhythm or position can be observed and noted. He should then be asked to squat, keeping his heels flat on the ground, and if the movement is full range and pain free he should next be asked to bounce up and down in this position so as to put maximum strain on to his foot.

The following tests are not strictly quick tests but they are informative functional tests which can be performed quickly and which will give the physiotherapist information as to whether pain or restriction is the dominant factor and where this pain or stiffness is largely occurring or is likely to occur.

1. The patient should be asked to walk normally, away from and then towards the physiotherapist. He should then be asked to walk backwards, away from and then towards the physiotherapist.
2. He should be asked to walk on his toes, towards the physiotherapist and then backwards away from her.
3. He should be asked to walk forwards and backwards, away from and towards, the physiotherapist, while on his heels and maintaining full dorsiflexion.
4. He should be asked to hop on the toes of his bad foot, and then on the heel of his bad foot keeping the ball of the foot well clear of the floor.

SPECIAL TESTS

The special tests involved in examining the patient's foot merely require the isolating of painful and/or restricted movements to the different joints which make up the foot so as to know where to emphasize the treatment techniques.

Table 8.8 outlines the objective examination for the intertarsal joints but some points need clarification. The tendon sheaths should be examined as a source of pain by performing resisted movements through a full range, making the tendon slide within the sheath. The 'differentiating' referred to in relation to dorsiflexion, plantar flexion, inversion and eversion means that these movements are first performed as full range passive movements for the total foot. If a movement is found to be painful or stiff, the general foot movement should be broken down into its different components so as to determine in which joint or joints the fault lies. For example, inversion includes inversion of the ankle and subtalar joints, adduction and rotation (sometimes called supination) which take place in all joints between the transverse tarsal joint and the tarsometatarsal joints, and finally plantar flexion at all joints. For example, it is possible to assess both range and pain caused by transverse tarsal rotation by grasping around the talus and calcaneus with one hand (so as to prevent them moving) while the other hand holds around the navicular and cuboid bones to rotate (supinate) them. Similar tests are done for the remaining movements. If inversion is painful or stiff, each component can be assessed separately.

Table 8.8
Intertarsal Joints: Objective Examination

Observation

Active tests (including quick tests)

Static tests

Other structures in 'plan'
　　Full active resisted movements through range for 'sheaths'

Passive movements
Physiological movements
　　Routinely
　　　　Differentiating DF, and PF, Inv, Ev
　　　　Note range, pain, resistance, spasm and behaviour
　　As applicable
　　　　The injuring or aggravating movements
Accessory movements
　　Routinely
　　　　For foot, differentiating intertarsal joints
　　　　1. Ab, Ad
　　　　2. ↻ ↺
　　　　3. HF and HE forefoot proximally. Differentiating
　　　　4. ↕ , ↑ , →•→, •→•, ↕ varying positions and angles
　　　　Note range, pain, resistance, spasm and behaviour

Palpation
　　Include tendon sheaths

Check case records etc.

HIGHLIGHT MAIN FINDINGS WITH ASTERISKS

After treatment

TECHNIQUES

Inversion**

Starting position

The patient lies prone with his knee flexed to a right angle and the physiotherapist stands by his right knee with her left knee on the couch to support his right shin. When the technique is used generally

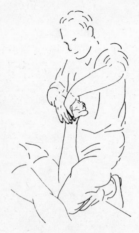

Figure 8.69. – Intertarsal movement, inversion; grades II and III–

for the whole foot she holds his foot with both hands from the lateral side, with her thumbs across the dorsum and her fingers across the plantar surface to reach the medial side (*Figure 8.69*).

Method

The physiotherapist moves the patient's foot away from her by laterally rotating his hip so that his lower leg moves through an arc of 15–20 degrees. To perform a large amplitude inversion movement she pulls the patient's foot towards her with her arms and simultaneously inverts his foot with her hands. She times the movements so that the swing of his leg assists her reaching the limit of inversion.

The movement may be performed in varying positions of dorsi-plantar flexion as dictated by the signs found on examination.

If III+ movements are required, a more economical starting position should be adopted.

GRADE III+**

The technique is still being performed as a general movement for the whole foot.

Starting position

The patient lies prone with his feet near the end of the couch. The physiotherapist, standing at the foot of the couch, holds his forefoot in both hands with her thumbs and thenar eminences along the sole

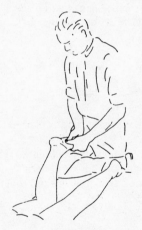

*Figure 8.70. – Intertarsal movement,
inversion; grade III+*

of the forefoot while her fingers overlap on the dorsum of the foot. She lifts his foot from the couch by flexing his knee, and places her right knee on the couch. She then lowers his leg, medially rotating his hip and inverting his foot, to rest his fully inverted foot against her thigh (*Figure 8.70*).

Method

The movement is difficult to perform well unless care is taken. Concentration should be centred around feeling the inversion/eversion movement right up to the limit of the range. It is an extremely effective and useful treatment technique.

From the starting position described above where the patient's fully inverted foot rests against her thigh, two movements take place. Firstly, the physiotherapist's arms move the patient's lower leg in a straight line, lifting his foot diagonally 18 inches away from her knee towards his opposite hip. This involves flexion of his knee and lateral rotation of his hip. The second movement is eversion of his foot combined with slight dorsiflexion, and this is performed by her hands. The return movement is also a combination of two movements but now they are the opposite of those described above. The inversion and plantar flexion movement is assisted by the drop of the lower leg and reaches the limit of the range when his foot reaches her thigh.

Because the physiotherapist grasps the metatarsals and has her thumb tips over their bases more movement takes place distal to the transverse tarsal joint than proximal to it. More rotation (supination) and plantar flexion take place also.

If IV+ movements are required a completely different technique is used.

GRADE IV+*

Two positions are shown for this technique. The first utilizes the whole foot with the emphasis on movement distal to the transverse tarsal joint and the second localizes the movement more to the hind foot, that is the talocrural and subtalar joints.

Starting position (No. 1)

The patient lies on his left side with his hips and knees comfortably flexed. His right foot extends to the end of the couch and the physiotherapist, standing behind his foot, places her left hand between the medial side of his foot and the edge of the couch to form a fulcrum for the inversion movement. She places the heel of her right hand directed distally, over the lateral border of the lateral two tarsometatarsal joints with her fingers directed distally over the plantar surface and her thumb over the dorsal surface. If necessary she places her left forearm against his lower leg laterally to prevent his knee lifting during the mobilization (*Figure 8.71*).

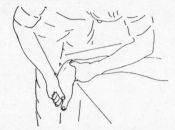

Figure 8.71. – Intertarsal movement, inversion; grade IV+ (starting position No. 1)

Method

Small amplitude oscillations performed strongly at the limit of the range are produced by direct pressure against the lateral border of the patient's foot. Small variations can be made in the position of the physiotherapist's hands and the direction of her pressure to produce maximum stretch in the appropriate direction and to localize the emphasis of the movement to a joint or functional group of joints.

Starting position (No. 2)

To localize the inversion (or adduction) to the talocrural joint and to the subtalar joint the physiotherapist uses the heel of her left hand against the lateral surface of the calcaneum while her right hand stabilizes the patient's metatarsals (*Figure 8.72*).

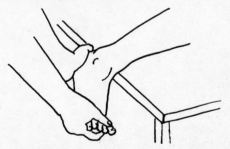

Figure 8.72. – Intertarsal movement, inversion; grade IV+ (starting position No. 2)

Method

Strong inversion can be produced by exerting pressure through the left hand, making use of the fingers to ensure that it is inversion which is being produced and not a medially directed transverse movement of the subtalar joint. This position can be used for strong oscillatory grade IV+ movements or, if indicated, the joints can be manipulated in this position.

Eversion**

As with inversion, described above, the following describes eversion as a general mobilizing technique. It, too, can be localized in the manner described above.

Starting position

The patient lies prone with his right knee flexed to a right angle while the physiotherapist stands by his knee with her left knee on the couch to support his right shin. She holds his whole foot from the lateral side with both hands. Her thumbs grasp over the dorsum of the foot and her fingers spread over the plantar surface reaching the medial longitudinal arch (*Figure 8.73*).

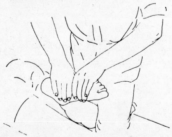

Figure 8.73. — Intertarsal movement, eversion; grades II and III—

Method

The technique for eversion is the same as that described for inversion (*see* page 290) except that it is movement of the patient's foot away from the physiotherapist which is the important part of the swinging action. This movement of his leg away from her needs to be carefully judged to assist the eversion of his foot performed by her hands.

If full range grade III+ type movements are required a more suitable starting position can be used.

GRADE III+**

Starting position

The patient lies prone with his feet reaching the end of the couch. The physiotherapist, standing at the foot of the couch, holds the patient's foot in both hands with her thumbs grasping over the plantar surface of

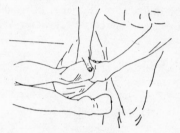

Figure 8.74. – Intertarsal movement, eversion; grade III+

the metatarsals and her fingers over the dorsal surface. She raises his foot and places her right knee on the couch near his left shin. She then lowers his foot, laterally rotating his hip and everting his foot to rest his lower leg and fully everted foot on her thigh (*Figure 8.74*).

Method

As was stated with the comparable technique for inversion (*see* page 291), though this technique is difficult to perform well, it is very effective treatment when used in the right circumstances. Two movements are coordinated. Firstly, the patient's knee is flexed and his hip medially rotated so that his foot traverses a straight line diagonally upwards and outwards. Secondly, the physiotherapist inverts his foot with her hands. The return movement combines dropping his leg towards her thigh, with eversion of the foot. The combined movement should be timed so that full eversion is reached when the patient's foot reaches her thigh.

When strong stretching movements are required in treatment a new position must be adopted.

GRADE IV+***

Starting position

The patient lies on his right side with his hips and knees comfortably flexed so that the lateral surface of his lower leg lies on the couch and his foot extends over the end of the couch. The physiotherapist stands behind his foot and positions her right hand between his foot and the edge of the couch to act as a comfortable fulcrum for the movement.

If the technique is to be performed as a general eversion of the whole foot then the physiotherapist places her right hand between the lateral malleolus and the edge of the couch. However, if on examination it

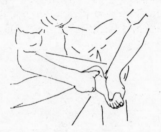

*Figure 8.75. – Intertarsal movement,
eversion, grade IV+*

has been possible to localize the painful or stiff joint during eversion, then she places the index finger of her right hand between that particular joint and the edge of the couch. With her left hand, if the eversion is to be performed as a general technique, she holds around the medial border of the foot around the metatarsals. If the technique is to be localized as referred to above, then she still holds around the medial border of the foot but localizes the technique by placing the heel of her left hand, through which most of the movement is transmitted, over the base of the first metatarsal, the medial cuneiform, the navicular bone or the talus.

She may need to position her right forearm across his leg to prevent it from lifting during the mobilization (*Figure 8.75*).

Method

Small amplitude oscillations produced firmly at the limit of the range
are imparted to the foot through the physiotherapist's left arm. During
the procedure she must modify the position of her hands and his foot
in relation to the fulcrum so that the leverage is economical and the
direction appropriate.

Abduction***

Abduction in this instance refers to abduction of the metatarsals and
intertarsal joints, about a vertical axis, and in relation to a stationary
talus and calcaneus.

Starting position

The patient lies prone with his knee flexed to a right angle while the
physiotherapist, standing by his knee facing his feet, places her left
knee on the couch to support his shin. She holds his foot around the
lateral border in both hands and places the pads of both thumbs over
the appropriate bones (*Figure 8.76*).

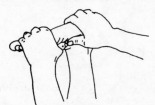

Figure 8.76. – Intertarsal movement;
abduction

This movement can be localized to the tarsometatarsal joint line,
or the calcaneocuboid joint laterally by placing the tip of her left
thumb over the tuberosity of the fifth metatarsal and the tip of her
right thumb over the cuboid bone. When the movement is localized to
the calcaneocuboid joint the tips of the thumbs are moved slightly
proximally to overlie adjacent lateral borders of the cuboid and the
calcaneus at the calcaneocuboid joint. During abduction the talo-
calcaneonavicular joint, the calcaneocuboid joint, the cuneonavicular
joint, cuboideonavicular joint, and intercuneiform and cuneocuboid
joints also move. By altering the positions of the thumb tips, the
movement can be emphasized at each joint.

Method

Small amplitude movements are produced by the physiotherapist's arms transmitting pressure through her thumbs while her encompassing grasp holds the patient's foot firmly. The action should not be produced by the muscles of the hand but should derive from an adduction of the shoulders which approximates the elbows. It is important that the movement should not be produced by a squeezing action of the hands. To do so would make the technique uncomfortable to the patient and the physiotherapist would lose all sense of feel of movement.

Adduction**

Adduction in this context relates to adduction of the metatarsals and tarsal bones anterior to the transverse tarsal joint around a vertical axis through the neck of the talus (*Figure 8.77*).

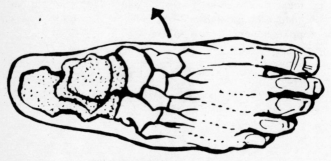

Figure 8.77. — Forefoot adduction

Starting position

The patient lies prone near the left edge of the couch with his right knee flexed. The physiotherapist stands by his left hip and holds his right foot from the medial aspect with both hands, placing the pads of her thumbs over the appropriate bones (*Figure 8.78*).

To localize or emphasize the adduction movement at the tarso-metatarsal joints, the physiotherapist places her right thumb over the base of the first metatarsal laterally and the tip of her left thumb over the medial cuneiform bone. To localize the movement to the navicular-medial cuneiform joint the thumbs are moved proximally to contact the navicular and medial cuneiform respectively. Similarly, to localize or emphasize the movement to the talonavicular joint the thumbs should be moved further proximally to lie over the talus and navicular

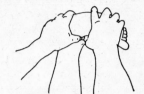

Figure 8.78. – Intertarsal movement; adduction

immediately adjacent to the joint line. As was described with abduction, when the adduction movement is performed, movement also takes place at the other intertarsal joints distal to the transverse tarsal joint.

Method

During this technique care must be taken to prevent the foot inverting and supinating.

As with the preceding technique, adduction must be performed by arm action and not by the thumbs. It is necessary to adjust the position of the patient's foot in relation to both dorsiplantar flexion and inversion/eversion to produce the adduction movement which is stiff or painful.

Plantar flexion***

Plantar flexion of the ankle joint has already been described (*see* page 275). The intertarsal joints are also capable of plantar flexion but it is difficult to completely isolate them individually.

Starting position

The patient lies prone with his knee flexed to a right angle while the physiotherapist, standing by his knee, places her left knee on the couch to support his shin. She holds his calcaneus in her right hand with the heel of her hand posteriorly, her fingers over the plantar surface of his calcaneus and her finger tips level with the transverse tarsal joint.

With her left hand she holds over the dorsal surface of his forefoot with her fingers reaching the medial border of the foot (*Figure 8.79*).

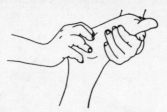

Figure 8.79. – Intertarsal movement;
plantar flexion

To localize the movement more finely a starting position similar to that described on page 299 (*Figure 8.78*) may be used. The point of difference between the two starting positions is that for plantar flexion the tips of the thumbs are placed on the plantar surfaces of each bone forming one of the intertarsal joints.

Method

While she holds his heel partly dorsiflexed she plantar flexes his forefoot with her left hand around the fulcrum of her right finger tips. She times her movement so that her right index finger can apply an equal and opposite counterpressure to that exerted by her left hand.

When it is desired to localize the movement to the joint mentioned in the starting position above, the oscillatory movement is created by an ulnar deviation of both wrists combined with glenohumeral adduction. Each hand should hold its part of the foot so that it moves as a single unit. The tips of the thumbs must be made to sink gradually through the soft tissue of the plantar surface of the foot until they can feel the plantar surfaces of the respective bones. They then form the fulcrum of the plantar flexion.

Dorsiflexion***

Dorsiflexion of the ankle has already been described (*see* page 277) but some dorsiflexion takes place also at the intertarsal joints.

Starting position

The patient lies prone, with his right knee flexed to a right angle, while the physiotherapist stands by his knee and places her left knee on the couch to support his shin. She holds the medial side of his calcaneus and talus in her right hand so that her fingers lie anterior to his ankle with her index finger over the transverse tarsal joint. Her right thenar eminence lies across the plantar surface of his calcaneus. She holds his forefoot in her left hand so that the thenar eminence lies over the plantar surface of the metatarsals and the palmar surface of the distal two phalanges of the index finger lie over the dorsal surface of the appropriate tarsal bone or bones (*Figure 8.80*).

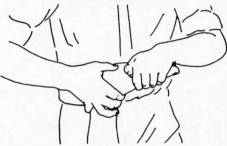

Figure 8.80. – Intertarsal movement; dorsiflexion

A different starting position, similar to that described for intertarsal abduction (page 297, *Figure 8.76*) can be used to localize or emphasize the movement at different intertarsal joints. The tips of the thumbs can be placed on the dorsal surfaces of the talus, the navicular, the calcaneus, the cuboid and the cuneiform bones, each in turn.

Method

While the physiotherapist's right hand holds the patient's heel plantar flexed she dorsiflexes his forefoot from a position of plantar flexion, endeavouring to apply an equal and opposite counterpressure with her right index finger.

When the technique is being used more specifically at each intertarsal joint the movement is produced by the physiotherapist's wrists and shoulders. Her fingers and thumb encompass the bones proximal and distal to the particular joint so that each hand and its bone moves as a single unit about the fulcrum formed by the thumbs at the intertarsal joint.

Postero-anterior and anteroposterior movements***

Only anteroposterior movement is depicted in *Figure 8.81*. It is unnecessary to describe postero-anterior movement as it is self-explanatory.

Starting position

The patient lies supine with his hip and knee flexed so that his foot can rest comfortably and flat on the couch. The physiotherapist stands at his feet, facing his head, and places the tips of her thumbs in the appropriate position over the dorsal surface of each tarsal bone in turn. Her fingers wrap comfortably around the foot to maintain stability (*Figure 8.81*).

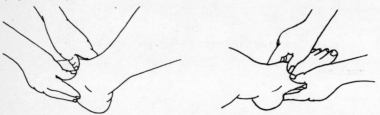

Figure 8.81. – Intertarsal anteroposterior movement

Method

Anteroposterior movements (and postero-anterior movements) of each tarsal bone are produced by the physiotherapist's arms and trunk, and are transmitted to the bones via the tips of the thumbs. Concentric intrinsic muscle action must not be used to produce the movement as this removes all possibility of the physiotherapist appreciating the movement of one bone, say the middle cuneiform bone, in relation to the adjacent bone or bones, in this case the other two cuneiform bones, the navicular and the metatarsal bone.

It must be remembered that the direction of the anteroposterior movement (or postero-anterior movement) may be varied within a dome, that is, it can be performed in combination with medial, lateral, cephalad or caudad inclinations. It must also be remembered that the tips of the thumbs may make contact directly over the joint line, directly over the proximal bone, directly over the distal bone, or over the medial or lateral bone (*see Figures 2.3–2.5*, page 23).

Gliding movements***

These movements were described in Chapter 2 on 'Examination' (*see Figures 2.1* and *2.2*, page 22). They consist of holding one tarsal bone between the fingers and thumb of one hand while holding the adjacent tarsal bone with which it forms a joint in the fingers and thumb of the other hand. The physiotherapist then holds one bone stationary and moves the adjacent bone in line with the joint surface.

TARSOMETATARSAL JOINT

Flexion and extension of the big toe are the only techniques which will be described as the remainder are identical in principle, although the grips vary. The 'quick tests' for these joints are the same as those described for the ankle and intertarsal joints. There are no particular 'special tests' relevant in this area. The examination is presented in Table 8.9.

Table 8.9
Tarsometatarsal Joints: Objective Examination

Observation

Active movements
> Active quick tests
> *Routinely*
> Gait, heel and toe walking forwards and backwards, hopping on toes, squatting on toes and flat feet
> DF, PF, Inv, Ev, toe F and E
> Note range and pain

Static tests

Other structures in 'plan'
> Full active resisted movements through range for 'sheaths'
> Joint restriction c.f. muscle/tendon restriction

Passive movements
Physiological movements
> *Routinely*
> F and E of toes, foot Inv, Ev, PF, DF
> Note range, pain, resistance, spasm and behaviour
Accessory movements
> *Routinely*
> ↕ ↑ ↕ (varying angles), →← ←← (with Ab and Ad),
> ↻ ↺ (with and without compression)
> HF and HE (general and local)
> Note range, pain, resistance, spasm and behaviour

Palpation
> Include tendon sheaths

Check case records etc.

HIGHLIGHT MAIN FINDINGS WITH ASTERISKS

After treatment

TECHNIQUES

Flexion***

Starting position

The patient lies prone with his knee flexed to a right angle and the physiotherapist stands by his knee. She places her left knee on the couch to support his shin. She holds the tarsometatarsal joint in both hands with the thumbs on the plantar surface of the adjacent bones at the joint and the index fingers around the medial border of the foot to support the joint on each side dorsally. The fingers of each hand support the remainder of the dorsum of the foot (*Figure 8.82*).

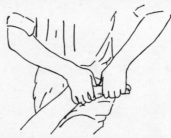

Figure 8.82. – Tarsometatarsal flexion

Method

The mobilization is produced by the physiotherapist's arms pivoting her fingers around her thumbs. As with all techniques in which the thumbs are used to produce movement, the thumb flexors must not be the prime movers. This technique is very effective if care is taken to localize the movement to the appropriate joint. In the presence of marked tenderness a larger area of the pad of the thumb should be used.

Extension***

Starting position

The patient lies prone with his knee flexed to a right angle and the physiotherapist stands by his knee. She places her left knee on the couch to support his shin and holds his foot around the medial border in both hands placing her index fingers, pointing laterally, across the dorsal surface of the adjacent bones at the joint. Her fingers spread over the adjacent dorsum of the foot while her left palm and thenar eminence hold the ball of the foot and her right palm and thenar eminence hold the plantar surface near the heel. She places her left thenar eminence over the plantar surface of the head of the metatarsal and her right hand around the medial and plantar surfaces of the tarsal bones (*Figure 8.83*).

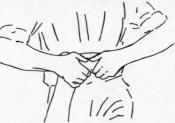

Figure 8.83. – Tarsometatarsal extension

Method

The mobilization is produced by an arm action which pivots the heel of each hand (particularly that of the left hand) around the fulcrum of the index finger. The right hand provides pressure at the tarsometatarsal joint rather than providing much in the way of movement.

Alternative method

The patient lies supine and flexes his hip and knee so that his foot lies comfortably flat upon the couch. Extension at each tarsometatarsal joint can be produced by placing the tips of the thumbs over the adjacent bones forming each intertarsal joint and using the leverage provided by the physiotherapist's fingers on the plantar surface of the patient's foot (*Figure 8.84*).

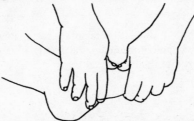

Figure 8.84. – Tarsometatarsal extension;
alternative method

This can also be done with the patient lying prone. The technique is similar to that shown in *Figure 8.76* (page 297).

Accessory movements

The movements now to be described are passive accessory movements which can be used both in examination and treatment. It should be appreciated that they can be combined together to produce a single accessory movement, or combined with the physiological movement of flexion or extension.

TRANSVERSE MOVEMENT**

As was described for the carpometacarpal joints, the tips of the thumbs can be placed against the base of each metatarsal to produce a transverse movement of the head of the metatarsal at the tarsometatarsal junction. The appropriate phalanges are used to assist the medial or lateral movement of the head of the metatarsal and the medial or lateral border of the foot is held by the physiotherapist's fingers to form a stable base about which the transversely directed pressure can be applied.

POSTERO-ANTERIOR AND ANTEROPOSTERIOR MOVEMENTS**

By placing the tips of the thumbs over the base of a metatarsal, either on the dorsal surface or the plantar surface, an anteroposterior or postero-anterior movement of the base of the metatarsal in relation to its adjacent tarsal bone is produced.

Again it is pointed out that these pressures in relation to the tarsometatarsal joints may be varied in their direction throughout a global sphere, and the pressures directed through the metatarsal, the adjacent tarsal bone or the joint line.

ROTATION***

Rotation is easily produced at the tarsometatarsal joints by flexing the metatarsophalangeal and interphalangeal joints of the toe and using this flexed toe to rotate the metatarsal.

GLIDING***

As with other joints in the hand and foot, it is possible to produce gliding movements at the tarsometatarsal joints by holding the appropriate cuneiform or cuboid bone in one hand, and the base of the metatarsal in the other hand, then moving the adjacent bones in opposite directions in line with the joint surface.

INTERMETATARSAL MOVEMENT

The intermetatarsal movements are anteroposterior and postero-anterior gliding, horizontal extension which flattens the foot across the heads of the metatarsals and horizontal flexion which increases the transverse arch of the foot. Postero-anterior and anteroposterior movements of one metatarsal in relation to its neighbour can be produced passively. The 'quick tests' have been described earlier with other joints of the foot, and the only 'special' test is horizontal flexion described below. Table 8.10 lists the examination.

Table 8.10
Intermetatarsal Movement: Objective Examination

Observation

Active movements

Static tests (not applicable)

Other joints in 'plan'

Passive movements
↕ individually (heads and bases)
HF and HE (and individually)
↓ and ↕ of each metacarpal in relation to its neighbours, varying the directions (heads and bases)
Note range, resistance, pain, spasm and behaviour

Palpation
Include tendon sheaths

Check case records etc.

HIGHLIGHT MAIN FINDINGS WITH ASTERISKS

After treatment

TECHNIQUES

Gliding***

Starting position

The patient lies prone with his feet near the end of the couch. The physiotherapist, standing at the foot of the couch, holds the distal end of the patient's metatarsals in both hands and flexes his knee slightly. She places her thumbs, pointing proximally, side by side over the plantar surface of two adjacent metatarsals and grasps the dorsal surface of each metatarsal with each flexed index finger in order to grasp the metatarsal between the index finger and thumb of each hand. She kneels with her right knee on the couch and supports her right hand against her right thigh (*Figure 8.85*).

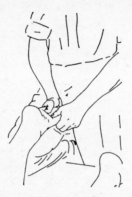

Figure 8.85. – Intermetatarsal movement;
gliding

Method

Each hand should hold the individual metatarsal firmly while the movement is produced by a pushing action with one hand countered by a pulling action with the other. The same technique is used whichever pair of metatarsals is mobilized.

Horizontal flexion*

Starting position

The patient lies prone with his feet near the end of the couch. The physiotherapist, standing at the foot of the couch, holds the patient's foot in her hands and flexes his knee slightly. By kneeling on her right knee, she can support her right hand against her thigh. She places the pads of her thumbs pointing towards each other over the plantar surface of the head of the third metatarsal while grasping around each side of the foot with her fingers. Her main finger contact is with the dorsal surface of the second and fourth metatarsals near their heads (*Figure 8.86*).

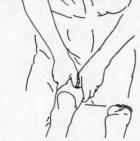

Figure 8.86. – Intermetatarsal movement;
horizontal flexion

Method

The horizontal flexion is produced by the physiotherapist's arms which, during adduction of the shoulders, pivot the fingers around the fulcrum of the thumbs. The examination findings may indicate that the movement should be pivoted around the second or fourth metatarsal rather than the third and this is achieved by placing the tips of the thumbs over the head of the relevant metatarsal.

Horizontal extension*

Starting position

The patient lies prone with his feet near the end of the couch. The physiotherapist, standing at the foot of the couch, holds the patient's foot in her hands and flexes his knee slightly. She places the metatarsal

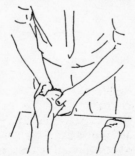

Figure 8.87. – Intermetatarsal movement;
horizontal extension

and phalanges of the thumb and thenar eminence of each hand, pointing towards his heel, over the plantar surface of the heads of the first and fifth metatarsals respectively. She places her fingers over the dorsum of the third metatarsal, using the pads of the fingers to make the contact more comfortable (*Figure 8.87*).

Method

The horizontal extension is produced by a supination action of the physiotherapist's forearms pivoting her thumbs around her fingers. As with the preceding technique, any of the metatarsals may be made the fulcrum of the movement.

Expertly assessing the behaviour of pain, resistance or muscle spasm in joints which make up the foot can be an exacting but interesting exercise. Table 8.11 lists the passive movement tests to be employed when a patient complains of pain or lacks normal function in his foot due to joint stiffness. It is a table showing the sequence of tests which are applied from the inferior tibiofibular joint proximally to the tarso-metatarsal joints distally.

Table 8.11
Composite Foot/Ankle: Objective Examination

Observation

Active quick tests
> Walking: forwards, backwards, on toes, on heels
> Balancing: on one leg
> Hopping: on flat foot, on toes, on heels
> Squatting: spontaneously; with heels on and off ground

Static tests

Other joints in 'plan'

Passive tests
Prone

Inferior tibiofibular joint
> ↕ , ↑ , compression, ↕ with compression, ↑ with compression

Whole foot
1. DF, PF; as IV−, to IV+, to III++
2. Inv, Ev; as IV−, to IV+, to III++
3. ↻ , ↺ , (axis in line with tibia) IV−, to IV+, to III++
4. ↔ ceph, caud, (axis in line with tibia) to III++
5. ↕ , ↑ , at ankle
6. Ab, Ad
7. HF, HE

Table 8.11 (cont.)

Differentiating as required
1. DF and PF as IV+ at limit of range
    (*a*) ankle (DF includes inferior tibiofibular movement)
    (*b*) transverse tarsal joint (talocalcaneonavicular and calcaneocuboid)
    (*c*) cuneonavicular
    (*d*) tarsometatarsal
2. Inv and Ev as IV+ at limit of range
    (*a*) inferior T/F joint
    (*b*) ankle (IV produces inferior T/F movement
    (*c*) subtalar (IV produces inferior T/F movement } Hind foot
    (*d*) transverse tarsal joint (talocalcaneonavicular and calcaneocuboid)
        (*i*)   rotation (i.e. Sup and Pron)
        (*ii*) Ab and Ad
        (*iii*) DF and PF
    (*e*) cuneonavicular
    (*f*) intercuneiform and cuneocuboid
        (*i*)   rotation, i.e. Sup and Pron
        (*ii*) Ab and Ad
        (*iii*) DF and PF
    (*g*) tarsometatarsal
        (*i*)   rotation, i.e. Sup and Pron
        (*ii*) Ab and Ad
        (*iii*) DF and PF
3. 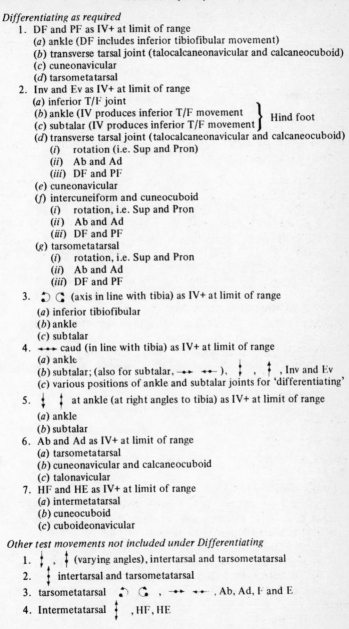 (axis in line with tibia) as IV+ at limit of range
    (*a*) inferior tibiofibular
    (*b*) ankle
    (*c*) subtalar
4. ←→ caud (in line with tibia) as IV+ at limit of range
    (*a*) ankle
    (*b*) subtalar; (also for subtalar, →→ ←→),   ↓ , ↑ , Inv and Ev
    (*c*) various positions of ankle and subtalar joints for 'differentiating'
5. ↓ ↑ at ankle (at right angles to tibia) as IV+ at limit of range
    (*a*) ankle
    (*b*) subtalar
6. Ab and Ad as IV+ at limit of range
    (*a*) tarsometatarsal
    (*b*) cuneonavicular and calcaneocuboid
    (*c*) talonavicular
7. HF and HE as IV+ at limit of range
    (*a*) intermetatarsal
    (*b*) cuneocuboid
    (*c*) cuboideonavicular

Other test movements not included under Differentiating
1. ↓ , ↑ (varying angles), intertarsal and tarsometatarsal
2. ↑ intertarsal and tarsometatarsal
3. tarsometatarsal ⟲ ⟳ , →→ ←→ , Ab, Ad, F and E
4. Intermetatarsal ↑ , HF, HE

Table 8.11 (cont.)

Palpation

Check case records etc.

HIGHLIGHT MAIN FINDINGS WITH ASTERISKS

After treatment

TREATMENT

The treatment of foot pain or stiffness is quickest and most successful when passive movements are localized to the precise directions of movement of the joint at fault. In most instances it is necessary to use the movements which reproduce the patient's pain or which produce a comparable pain at an appropriate joint. Although general movements, for example full inversion of the whole foot, can be used in treatment, the result will be achieved more quickly if the comparable sign can be isolated to a single joint's movement and if this movement is used as the treatment technique.

In the treatment of most joint pain problems of the foot, grade IV type movements are most commonly used, to increase pain-free range or to provoke a controlled degree of the patient's pain. Alternatively, grade III movements, where the joint or joints involved are moved back and forth through a large range of movement up to the limit of the range, may be applied.

METATARSOPHALANGEAL AND INTERPHALANGEAL JOINTS

EXAMINATION

Table 8.12 lists the examination for these joints. The 'quick tests' are squatting, gait tests and hopping as listed in Table 8.7.

The movements which can be performed at the metatarsophalangeal and interphalangeal joints are identical with those of the fingers described on pages 187–197. Compression is an important component which, as a 'special test' may be added to any test movement of the metatarsophalangeal and interphalangeal movements.

Table 8.12
Metatarsophalangeal and Interphalangeal Joints: Objective Examination

Observation

Active movements
    Active quick tests
    Gait, walking on toes forwards and backwards, hopping, squatting on heels
    and toes
    As applicable
    The injuring or aggravating movements

Static tests

Other structures in 'plan'
    Joint restriction c.f. muscle/tendon restriction

Passive movements
Physiological movements
    Routinely
        F and E of toes
        Note range, pain, resistance, spasm and behaviour
Accessory movements
    Routinely
       1. $\uparrow$, $\downarrow$, $\longrightarrow$, $\longleftarrow$, Ab, Ad, $\supset$, $\subset$, $\longleftrightarrow$ ceph and caud (with and
          without compression
       2. Above techniques combined in varying sequences
       3. For metatarsophalangeal joints add HF and HE, general and localized
       Note range, pain, resistance, spasm and behaviour

Palpation
    Include tendon sheaths

Check case records etc.

HIGHLIGHT MAIN FINDINGS WITH ASTERISKS

After treatment

TECHNIQUES

Abduction of the metatarsophalangeal joint of the big toe is shown in *Figure 8.88*. It is frequently of value in the treatment of hallux valgus. Under these circumstances abduction is used as grade IV and grade III—movements.

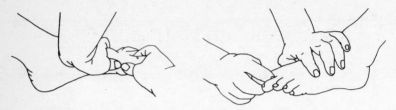

Figure 8.88. – Metatarsophalangeal abduction of the big toe

The big toe frequently requires mobilizing in many or all directions and compression is very often required in conjunction with such movements as abduction or rotation. The techniques can be carried out with the patient supine or prone. However, the prone position with the patient's knee flexed to a right angle and supported is one which is most economical for the physiotherapist and one which assists relaxation to a surprising degree.

TREATMENT

The metatarsophalangeal joints of one or more toes are very frequently the source of what is diagnosed as 'metatarsalgia'. Localized mobilizing techniques of the joint are very effective as well as producing quick results.

9 Other Joints and Structures

COSTAL JOINTS AND INTERCOSTAL MOVEMENT

Symptoms arising from the musculoskeletal structures of the thorax area usually have a traumatic origin and passive movement treatment can frequently be used with good effect. Synovial joints exist in the costochondral, interchondral and sternocostal articulations. Even though there are no intercostal joints, the movement between the ribs can be restricted and painful. As with the sternoclavicular joint (*see Figures 6.39* and *6.40),* the direction of movement can be varied to suit the findings on examination. Movement in only one direction will be described but reference will be made to movement in other directions. The 'quick test' involves maximum inspiration (and expiration) and inspiration performed at maximum speed (Table 9.1).

Table 9.1
Costal Joints and Intercostal Movement: Objective Examination

Observation

Active movements
> *Active quick tests*
>> Inspiration, max and quickly (expiration)
> *Routinely*
>> Trunk F, E, LF, Rot.[n]
>> Note range and pain
> *As applicable*
>> The injuring or aggravating movements

315

Table 9.1 (cont.)

Static tests

Other joints in 'plan'

Passive movements
Physiological movements
   Routinely
      As for routine active movements above with overpressure
Accessory movements
   ↕ ↕   →• •← , adding ceph and caud and other varying angles
      Note range, pain, resistance, spasm and behaviour

Palpation
      For intercostal spacing, prominence and thickening

Check case records etc.

HIGHLIGHT MAIN FINDINGS WITH ASTERISKS

After treatment

Anteroposterior movement***

Starting position

The physiotherapist stands by the patient's right shoulder facing
across his trunk. To increase intercostal movement she places the pads
of her thumbs side by side across the joint to be mobilized with her
fingers spreading in a fan to provide stability. As much of the pad as

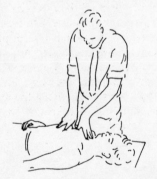

*Figure 9.1. – Costal joints and intercostal
movement; anteroposterior movement*

possible is used to make the contact more comfortable. The thumbs are more stable in this position than when directed along the shaft of the rib. She must position her shoulders directly above her hands and keep the base of her thumbs close together (*Figure 9.1*).

When symptoms can be attributed to abnormal movement between adjacent ribs the thumbs are placed along the line of the rib to spread the pressure area on the ribs. The physiotherapist directs her arms cephalad or caudad so that the movement will stretch the restriction or reproduce the symptoms.

Method

As with all other techniques involving the use of the thumbs, the anteroposterior movement must be produced by trunk and arm movements rather than by the thumb flexors.

The mobilization may be directed towards the patient's feet by applying pressure against the upper border of the rib. The physiotherapist then stands alongside the patient's head. If the movement is to be directed in an upward direction with the contact against the lower border of the rib, she must stand by the patient's right side at waist level. In both of these positions the thumbs may be directed along the shaft of the rib.

LARYNGEAL AND HYOID JOINTS

Synovial joints occur in pairs between the inferior cornua of the thyroid cartilage and the sides of the cricoid cartilage and also between the facets on the lateral surfaces of the upper border of the lamina of the cricoid cartilage and the base of the arytenoid cartilage. Occasionally there is a synovial joint between the lesser cornua and the greater cornua in the hyoid bone. It is not common for pain to arise from these joints but as they are synovial joints and are supported by ligaments they can, and in fact occasionally do, give rise to symptoms.

Coughing and swallowing are the only active 'quick tests'. The passive movement test consists of holding the adjacent cartilages with the index finger and thumb of each hand so as to be able to produce transverse and rotary movements.

Starting position*

The patient lies without a pillow so that neither his head nor his neck are flexed. The physiotherapist loosely grasps the upper and lower margins of the thyroid cartilage between the index finger and thumb of her left and right hands respectively. Her fingers spread forward over the adjacent neck, chest and face with her little fingers making the firmest contact (*Figure 9.2*).

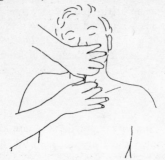

Figure 9.2. – Thyroid cartilage movement

Method

Movement of the thyroid cartilage away from the physiotherapist is produced by pressure through the thumbs. The little fingers form a pivot about which the thumb movement takes place. To make the pressure as comfortable as possible the movement should be produced by glenohumeral adduction and slight elbow extension rather than by the thumb flexors. Movement of the thyroid cartilage towards the physiotherapist is produced by the opposite movement of her arms acting through her index fingers. A rotary movement can also be performed.

Movement of the hyoid bone in relation to the mandible and thyroid cartilage can be produced by holding the hyoid bone between the index finger and thumb of the left hand while stabilizing the thyroid cartilage with the right hand.

TEMPOROMANDIBULAR JOINT

Movements of the jaw include depression, elevation, protraction, retraction, lateral movements of the chin, and the accessory postero-anterior and transverse movements and longitudinal movement cephalad and caudad of the head of the mandible.

EXAMINATION

Alignment of teeth during opening and closing of the mouth is important to watch as is the occlusal position. Subjectively it is important to determine whether the patient has pain during chewing or yawning (Table 9.2).

Table 9.2
Temporomandibular Joint: Objective Examination

Observation

Active movements
   Routinely
      Note occlusal position
      Depression, elevation, protraction, retraction; note range and straightness; lateral movement
      Note range and pain for all movements
      Muscle power
      Upper cervical spine

Static tests

Other joints in 'plan'

Passive movements
   Routinely
      Depression, elevation, protraction, retraction and lateral mandibular movements
      $\uparrow$, $\uparrow$, $\rightarrow$, $\leftarrow$, $\rightarrow$ ceph and caudad (with and without compression)
      Note range, pain, resistance, spasm and behaviour

Palpation
      Capsular thickening

Check case records etc.

HIGHLIGHT MAIN FINDINGS WITH ASTERISKS

After treatment

TECHNIQUES

One of the greatest difficulties encountered when passively mobilizing the jaw is the patient's inability to relax his jaw completely. This may be one of the reasons why mobilization using pressure against the head of the mandible is much more successful in the treatment of jaw pain than techniques which involve large movements of the mandible. The two accessory movements will be described first.

Transverse movement medially***

Starting position

The patient lies with his head turned to the left, resting on a pillow. The physiotherapist stands behind his head and places the pads of her thumbs pointing towards each other over the head of the mandible.

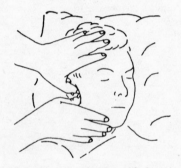

Figure 9.3. – Temporomandibular joint; transverse movement medially

She spreads her fingers comfortably around her thumbs to provide stability and positions the backs of her thumbs close together. Her arms must be directed in line with the transverse movement of the joint (*Figure 9.3*).

Method

Small amplitude oscillatory mobilizations are produced by her arms acting through her thumbs. Very little pressure is required to produce quite a lot of movement. Care must be exercised to make the technique as comfortable as possible.

Transverse movement laterally***

Starting position

The patient lies supine and the physiotherapist stabilizes his head with her left hand. She then places the pad of her right thumb, facing laterally against the medial surface of the ramus of the mandible, close to or against the head of the mandible (*Figure 9.4*).

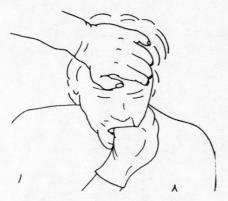

*Figure 9.4. – Temporomandibular joint;
transverse movement laterally*

Method

Gentle oscillatory pressures are applied to the medial surface of the mandible so as to produce lateral movement of the head of the mandible in the mandibular fossa of the temporal bone. The physiotherapist holds the ramus between her thumb, within the patient's mouth, and her fingers, outside the mouth on the lateral surface of the ramus. With this grasp the movement is produced by the action of the physiotherapist's arm, care being taken not to use the thumb flexors concentrically, but rather, eccentrically. If the technique is not performed in this manner the pressure on the medial surface of the ramus will be most uncomfortable.

The physiotherapist should also place the pad of one finger over the temporomandibular joint so that the range of lateral movement will be readily discernible.

Postero-anterior movement***

Starting position

The patient lies with his head turned to the left, resting on a pillow, or lies on his left side. The physiotherapist stands by his right shoulder and places the pads of her thumbs, pointing towards each other, against

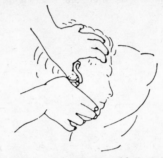

*Figure 9.5. – Temporomandibular joint;
postero-anterior movement*

the posterior surface of the head of the mandible, behind the lobe of the ear, with the backs of her thumbs close together. Her fingers rest comfortably over the head and jaw. She directs her forearms in line with the postero-anterior movement of the joint (*Figure 9.5*).

Method

Mobilization in this direction is produced by the physiotherapist's arms acting through her thumbs. As this area is normally tender, it is necessary to position the thumbs carefully and produce movement with the arms and not the thumb flexors.

Protraction**

Starting position

The patient lies with his head resting comfortably on a pillow. The physiotherapist stands beyond his head, facing his feet. She holds his mandible by placing her thumbs in his mouth with the medial border of her thumbs against the inner surface of his lower incisors and the posterolateral surface of the interphalangeal joints against the outer surface of his upper incisors. Her fingers grasp comfortably under either side of the mandible (*Figure 9.6*).

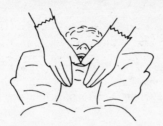

Figure 9.6. – Temporomandibular joint;
protraction

Method

Oscillatory protraction movements are produced by pivoting the tips of the thumbs against the lower teeth around the fulcrum of the interphalangeal joint against the upper teeth. This action should be produced by the physiotherapist's hand and forearm and not by the thumb flexors.

Retraction*

Starting position

The patient lies with his head resting on a pillow. The physiotherapist stands beyond his head, facing his feet. She places the pads of her thumbs, pointing towards his feet, against the anterior margin of the

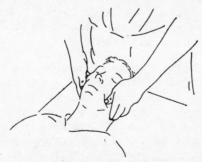

Figure 9.7. – Temporomandibular joint;
retraction

ramus of the mandible while her fingers reach comfortably around the side of his head. The base of the pad of her thumb makes the main contact, not the tip (*Figure 9.7*).

Method

The retraction is produced by the physiotherapist's arms acting through the base of her thumbs. Care must be taken to prevent the thumbs sliding laterally off the ramus by directing some pressure medially.

Lateral chin movement***

Starting position

The patient lies with his head turned to the left, resting on a pillow, while the physiotherapist stands behind his head. She places her left hand over the left zygomatic arch to stabilize his head, preventing it from rotating further to the left during the mobilization. She adopts a

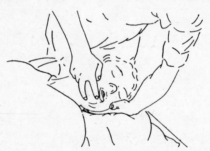

Figure 9.8. – Temperomandibular joint;
lateral chin movement

particular grasp of the right side of the mandible with her right hand so that she will be able to protract the right temporomandibular joint and displace the chin to the left. She places her index finger and thumb along the line of the jaw laterally and her middle finger beneath the jaw so that she can grasp it to control the opened or closed position of the mouth. Her ring and little fingers are flexed at the metacarpophalangeal and proximal interphalangeal joints so that the lateral border of the ring finger can be placed behind the angle of the jaw. The little finger reinforces the ring finger (*Figure 9.8*).

Method

With the patient's mouth slightly open and his jaw held firmly in the physiotherapist's right hand she produces movement of the jaw with her right hand. She should endeavour to pivot the right half of the jaw around the left temporomandibular joint.

Depression**

Starting position

The patient rests his head on a pillow while the physiotherapist stands by his right upper arm facing his head. She holds each side of his mandible in her hands so that the pads of her middle and ring fingers

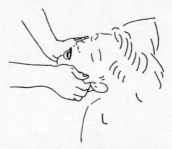

Figure 9.9. — Temporomandibular joint; depression

contact the posterior surface of the ramus of the mandible near the head. The metacarpophalangeal joint of the thumb and thenar eminence are placed against the superior margin of the body of the mandible near the chin. Care must be taken to use as much of the pads of the fingers as possible to make the contact comfortable (*Figure 9.9*).

Method

This movement must be produced by the physiotherapist's wrists and arms while her hands move with his jaw as a single unit. She can control the depression to encourage protraction of the head of the mandible or backward movement of the angle of the jaw. This is achieved by increasing the work performed through the fingers or that performed through the base of the thumbs because patients find relaxation so difficult. This is the most difficult of the techniques described for the jaw. However, by performing the movements smoothly and encouraging relaxation, a finely controlled movement can be performed.

ALTERNATIVE TECHNIQUE

Starting position

The patient lies supine and the physiotherapist places two fingers of each hand into his mouth so as to grasp over the upper and lower incisors (*Figure 9.10*).

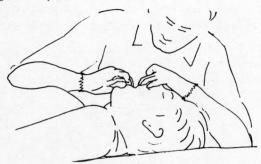

Figure 9.10. – Temporomandibular joint; depression. Alternative technique

Method

The physiotherapist stabilizes his maxilla with her left hand and applies oscillatory movements (usually at the limit of the range of depression) holding firmly with the fingers of her right hand while producing the movement with her right arm.

Longitudinal movement caudad**

Starting position

The patient lies supine and the physiotherapist places her right thumb in his mouth with the pad of her thumb facing caudad and braced against his lower left molars. She then stabilizes his head with her left hand (*Figure 9.11*).

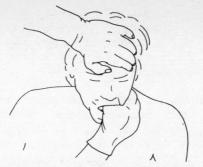

Figure 9.11. – Temporomandibular joint;
longitudinal movement caudad

Method

While stabilizing the patient's head with her left hand, the physiotherapist exerts pressure against his left lower molars so as to distract
the temporomandibular joint. This is best produced as an oscillatory
movement at the limit of the range, with the physiotherapist feeling
the extent of the joint movement by placing one finger of her right hand
over the lateral surface of the temporomandibular joint.

Longitudinal movement cephalad*

Starting position

The patient lies supine and the physiotherapist stabilizes his head
between her right hand and her thorax. She places the heel of her left
hand on the inferior margin of the angle of the mandible.

Method

The technique is one of pushing cephalad to jam the head of the
mandible against the articular disc and mandibular fossa.

TREATMENT

When a temporomandibular joint is locked, with the mouth fixed in
the open position, the best technique is one which combines caudad

longitudinal movement with repeated oscillatory depression and elevation rocking close to the point of limited elevation. An alternative procedure, also performed while the temporomandibular joint is held distracted, is either to rock the head of the mandible in an antero-posterior to postero-anterior direction or to rock it medially and laterally.

For the most part, patients seek treatment because they have pain in the region of their temporomandibular joint when chewing, biting with a widely opened mouth, or yawning. This pain usually responds very readily to medial transverse oscillatory movements (*see Figure 9.3,* page 320).

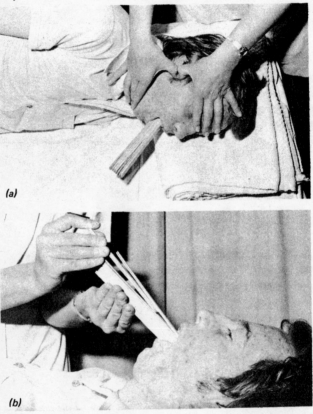

Figure 9.12. — (a) Transverse accessory movement at the limit of mandibular depression. (b) Inserting spatulas following mobilizing and 'contract/relax' techniques. (Reproduced by courtesy of P. H. Trott[1])

The third common disorder of this joint is one of very limited depression which prevents the patient from eating normally. The passive movement technique effecting depression has been described but if the condition is chronic, or the limitation of mandibular movement is severe, then the use of spatulas is necessary to maintain the range gained passively and to exercise the muscles producing depression by 'contract/relax' techniques. The complete treatment for this problem is described fully by P. H. Trott[1]. *Figure 9.12a* shows transverse pressure mobilizing being administered with the mouth opened at its maximum range by the use of spatulas. *Figure 9.12b* shows more spatulas being inserted following the mobilization described above and 'contract/relax' procedures.

This is a perfect example of the use of accessory movements at the limit of the range when treating joint stiffness as described in point 2 on page 50.

[1] Trott, P. H. (1976). 'Temporomandibular myofascial pain dysfunction syndrome'. Thesis for Graduate Diploma in Manipulative Therapy

Part III

APPLICATION

10 Recording

The need for care and attention to detail during continual assessment has been emphasized throughout the text. Once the patient has been examined a plan of treatment is made and the first technique is carried out. While it is being performed the physical signs of the joint should be watched and slight modifications to the technique may be made during the treatment if necessary. When the technique has been carried out for the necessary length of time the patient is asked to sit or stand so that a reassessment can be made. This reassessment may require some change in the plan of treatment. Perhaps a change of movement direction, perhaps the addition of a second direction or perhaps increasing the depth of the movement previously used. The changed treatment movement is then carried out. Each technique and its effect must be adequately recorded.

C/O

At the beginning of each treatment session the patient is asked to report any changes he feels as a result of treatment. To determine the exact effect of a session of treatment it should be established how the patient felt when the day's treatment was completed as compared with how he felt before treatment, whether he felt that his symptoms were any different the night following the treatment, and if there was any difference in his symptoms when he first arose the morning after treatment. The patient's spontaneous comments are the most useful guide and to provide the opportunity for these the physiotherapist may ask general questions first. It may then be necessary to ascertain more precisely the immediate effect of treatment, the effect it may have had during the night of treatment, and the effect it may have had the following morning. These findings are recorded first.

O/E

The subjective assessment should be followed by the physiotherapist's own assessment of the changes in the important movements to be measured, noting in particular any changes in the behaviour of the pain with active movements and in the range. Fine differences in pain pattern need to be sought before deciding whether a test movement is better or worse than when performed at the previous treatment session. For example, on re-examination, it may be found that pain still starts at the same point in the range and the movement is still limited by the pain at the same degree of movement. However, by watching the way the patient moves his joint, and by questioning, it may be determined that the pain now remains at a lower intensity in the early part of the painful range before sharply increasing to its maximum, whereas previously it may have been increasing more rapidly in intensity at the beginning of the painful range. In such an instance it can be considered that there has been improvement in this movement.

It should be appreciated that a patient may have two or more kinds of pain felt at one point or that he may have two different pains at two different places. When such circumstances exist changes in the type and site of pain should also be sought.

℞

Recording the treatment can be considered in two parts. The first part is recording the treatment movement used and its effect during treatment. The second is recording the effect of the treatment movement on the joint after it has been completed. These two parts should be sought separately. To separate them when recording by a short vertical line will enhance clarity of thinking and presentation. It also makes retrospective assessment quicker and clearer.

The vertical line is useful in that it highlights the treatment part of the record which assists easier review of progress over a period of treatment. It is often necessary to check back over treatment to assess whether a particular avenue has been explored or not, or to determine whether something different should be attempted. Whatever method of recording is used, the important fact is that an adequate record must be made during each treatment. The method suggested is realistic and does not occupy much time. To attempt treatment without some such routine is to invite bad treatment and poor results.

The treatment record on the left-hand side of the vertical line should include the following: (1) the joint treated; (2) the technique used; (3) the grade of movement used; (4) number of times done and (5) any effect felt by the patient while the technique was being carried out.

On the right-hand side of the vertical line which separates the description of the treatment from its effect, the following facts should be recorded: C/O — any change which the patient feels has taken place as a result of the treatment technique; and O/E — an assessment of changes which have taken place in the movements (Table 10.1).

Table 10.1
Recording Each Treatment During Treatment

C/O   *Subjective assessment.* Interpret what the patient says carefully. Check on any asterisked points. With patients whose progress can be expected to be slow, make the comparison over a week, as well as over 24 hours

O/E   *Objective assessment.* Check important signs which are asterisked

Plan   State why you choose a certain technique/exercises/heat

Treatment	Effect after ℞
℞ *State:*	
1. The joint being treated	C/O
2. The technique used	
3. The grade used	
4. The number of times it was done	
5. *The effect it had while being performed*	O/E

Plan   State reason for any change required and note any reminders for next treatment

Example

C/O   'Less shoulder pain, slept better'

O/E   F pain starts 100° (20° imp.) and can reach full range now

Plan   Is continuing to improve at anticipated rate, so repeat technique

℞		
1. ®G/H joint		C/O 'easier'
2. ↕ arm by side		
3. III –		
4. 3 X		O/E F pain starts 135°
5. No pain		

Plan   Satisfactory progress; probably continue rather than change to physio-logical movements

The treatment technique can be detailed yet brief, taking up little space, as a repeat of the above shows:

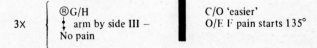

3X   ®G/H   C/O 'easier'
      ↕ arm by side III –   O/E F pain starts 135°
      No pain

Use must be made of abbreviations to describe the treatment techniques, and suggestions are given in Tables 10.2 and 10.3.

Table 10.2
Grades of Passive Movement

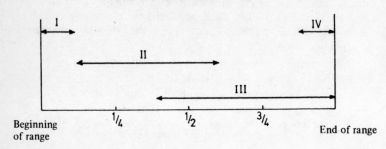

There are four grades of *mobilization*
I   small amplitude in beginning of range
II   large amplitude within the range
III   large amplitude up to the end of range
IV   small amplitude up to the end of range

There are two kinds of *manipulation*
V   small amplitude general movement performed quickly at end of range
ʄV   manipulation localized to a single joint movement in a multiple joint area (e.g. hand or foot)

Table 10.3
Symbols of Mobilization

F	Flexion
E	Extension
Ab	Abduction
Ad	Adduction
↻	Lateral rotation
↺	Medial rotation
Q	Quadrant
Lock	Locking position
F/Ab	Flexion abduction

Table 10.3 (cont.)

F/Ad	Flexion adduction
HF	Horizontal flexion
HE	Horizontal extension
Dist	Distraction
Comp	Compression
↕	Postero-anterior movement
↕	Anteroposterior movement
←•→	Longitudinal movement
	(a) ceph Cephalad
	(b) caud Caudad
—•→	Transverse movement in the direction indicated
↕	Gliding adjacent joint surfaces
Inv	Inversion
Ev	Eversion
DF	Dorsiflexion
PF	Plantarflexion
Sup	Supination
Pron	Pronation
EL	Elevation
DE	Depression
PR	Protraction
RE	Retraction
Med	Medial
Lat	Lateral

Appendix 1

Movement diagrams depict not only the pain and resistance found on joint examination but also their strength at different points in range: that is, they depict the behaviour of each throughout the range and in relation to each other. The response of the joint to movement is thus shown in a very detailed way. The value of the diagram lies in its use as a teaching aid and as a means of communication in technical discussion. The theory of the diagram is discussed here in its separate components, and Appendix 2 shows a step-by-step compilation of a diagram for one movement of one joint.

The joint disorder components discussed are pain and physical resistance to movement, with the latter being subdivided into the resistance offered by muscle activity such as spasm, and other kinds of resistance free from muscle activity such as capsular thickening or adhesions. Each of these three factors is an extensive subject, and it should be appreciated that the discussion is deliberately limited in various ways.

1. Discussion of pain is confined to pain felt at the site of the joint being examined; referred pain is not dealt with, though if the essence of the exercise is grasped it will be seen how the diagram can be extended to include this.

2. The spasm referred to is protective muscle spasm secondary to joint disorder; spasticity caused by upper motor neurone disease is excluded. So also is voluntary muscular contraction.

3. Resistance free of muscle activity is discussed only from the clinical point of view; discussion about pathology is excluded.

338

A movement diagram is compiled by drawing graphs depicting the behaviour of pain, spasm and physical resistance. The base line AB represents 'position in range' and 'intensity' of the factor is plotted on the vertical axis AC (*Figure A1.1*).

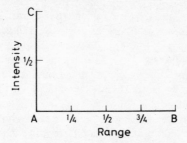

Figure A1.1. − Beginning the graph for
movement diagram

The base line AB represents any range of movement of any joint from the starting position at A to the limit of the normal range at B. It makes no difference whether the movement depicted is small or large, involves one joint or more than one joint, or represents the whole range or part of the range. For example, AB might represent one-eighth of an inch of sternoclavicular accessory movement or 200 degrees of glenohumeral scapulothoracic flexion.

Point B at the limit of normal range is always constant, but the starting position (point A) of the movement represented is variable. The position chosen might be the extreme of range opposite to B or a position somewhere in mid-range, whichever will represent the three factors best. For example, if elbow extension is the movement being represented, and pain or limitation occurs only in the last 10 degrees of the range, the diagram will more clearly demonstrate the findings if the base line represents the last 90 degrees of elbow extension rather than the last 160 degrees of elbow extension. However, if the elbow extension movement is restricted by 80 degrees or more, a base line representing the last 90 degrees would be inadequate; it would need to represent the last 160 degrees of elbow extension.

To make the diagram clear, the position should be defined by stating the range represented by the base line. In the above example, if the base line represents 160 degrees, A must be the position of full elbow flexion. Similarly if the base line represents the last 90 degrees, position A is with the elbow bent to a right angle.

Point B, representing the limit of normal range, does not vary. It must be clearly understood, however, that this point represents the extreme of passive movement, and that this lies variably, but importantly, somewhat beyond the extreme of active movement. For example, where the extreme of range depicted involves tissue approximation (as in flexion of the knee), or increasing tissue tension (as in extension of the metacarpophalangeal joint of the index finger), active range terminates approximately where passive movement encounters the first resistance of the tissues; the end of passive movement lies considerably further into the range, and is accompanied by a build-up of the resistance to movement. By contrast, in extension of the elbow the end of the range is defined by a hard bone-to-bone feel, encountered at almost the same point in range whether actively or passively. The feel of the resistance offered at the end of range is different in each of the examples given, but in each case the end of active range lies short of position B.

The vertical axis AC represents the intensity of the factors being plotted: point A represents absence of the factor, and C its maximum intensity. The meaning of maximum in relation to each factor needs defining and is discussed later in detail.

The basic diagram is completed by vertical and horizontal lines drawn from B and C to meet at D (*Figure A1.2*).

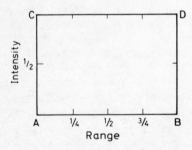

Figure A1.2. – Completion of the basic graph for movement diagram

PAIN

Examination for pain differs from the examination for physical resistance. Although in practice they are assessed at the same time, it is easier to establish their individual characteristics if they are considered separately in the first instance.

The first fact to be established is whether or not the patient has any pain while the joint is at rest; a joint which is pain free at rest is considered first.

The joint is moved slowly and carefully into the chosen range and the patient is asked to report immediately any discomfort. The position at which pain is first felt is not always easy to establish. Following a slow movement, during which the patient is asked to say when pain is first felt, several small slow oscillatory movements may be required to determine the exact point when pain starts. There is no danger of exacerbation if sufficient care is used and if the examiner appreciates that it is the very first provocation of pain which is being sought. The point at which this occurs is called P_1 and is marked on the base line of the diagram (*Figure A1.3*).

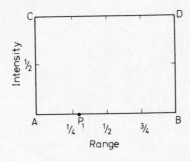

Figure A1.3. – Pain

The next step is to show how the pain behaves during movement into the painful range. To do this, the intensity of pain in any one position is assessed as lying somewhere between no pain at all and the maximum on the vertical axis of the graph (that is between A and C). It is important to realize that the maximum intensity of pain in the diagram represents the maximum amount of pain the physiotherapist is prepared to provoke. Naturally it is well within, and quite different from, a level which represents intolerable pain for the patient. Estimation of maximum in this way is entirely subjective and will vary with each physiotherapist.

The joint is moved slowly beyond P_1 while the patient is watched carefully to estimate change in pain. For example, very shortly beyond P_1 the intensity of pain may increase sharply so that the physiotherapist decides that no further movement should be attempted. This point of limitation in the range is marked on the base line as L which represents the limit of the available range. Since L represents the point at which pain becomes a limiting factor, that is, pain is of maximum intensity, the graph for pain appears as a line drawn from P_1 to intersect the upper horizontal CD at a position vertically above L. This point is called P_2 (*Figure A1.4*).

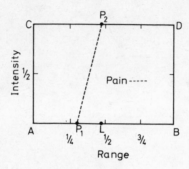

Figure A1.4. – Pain

Pain may not increase evenly in the way shown in *Figure A1.4*; its build-up may be irregular, calling for a graph which is curved or angular. For example, in *Figure A1.5a*, pain is first felt at about half range and increases quickly the further the movement is taken, reaching a limiting intensity at three-quarter range. In *Figure A1.5b*, pain is first felt at quarter range and remains at a low level until suddenly increasing in intensity, limiting movement at three-quarter range.

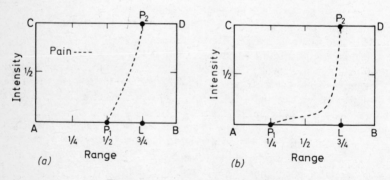

Figure A1.5. – Irregular increase of pain

The examples given have pain which limits movement of the joint, but instances occur where pain may never be so great as to limit range. For example, in *Figure A1.6*, a little pain is felt at half range but hardly increases at all beyond this point; the end of normal range is reached without provoking such intensity as would forbid further movement. There is thus no point L and P_2 appears on the vertical line BD.

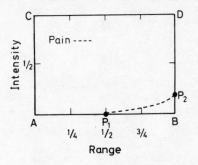

Figure A1 6. – Non-limiting pain

If we consider the joint which is painful at rest, an estimate must be made of the degree of pain present while the joint is at rest and this appears as P_1 on the vertical axis AC (*Figure A1.7a*). The joint is moved carefully until the pain begins to increase (X in *Figure A1.7a*).

The behaviour of pain beyond this point is plotted in the manner already described and an example of such a graph is given in *Figure A1.7b*.

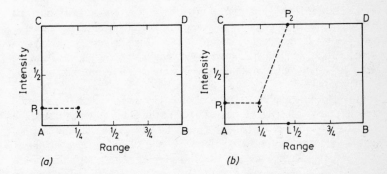

Figure A1.7. – (a) Pain in joint at rest; (b) pain due to subsequent movement

When the joint is painful at rest it must be appreciated that the symptoms are easily exacerbated by poor handling. However, if examination is carried out with sensitivity, no difficulty will be encountered.

It must again be emphasized that this evaluation of pain is purely subjective. Nevertheless, it presents an invaluable method of discerning the various ways pain can behave and students' appreciation of the subject will mature as this type of assessment is repeated from patient to patient and checked against the judgment of a more experienced physiotherapist.

PHYSICAL RESISTANCE

A normal joint, when completely relaxed and moved passively, has the feel of being well oiled and free running. It can be likened to wet soap sliding on wet glass.

If any resistance is encountered on examination of joint movement, an attempt must be made first to decide the type of resistance encountered and then to make a graph of its behaviour during movement in the same way as has been described for pain.

Resistance to movement is here divided into two types:

1. The resistance offered by muscle activity such as spasm; and
2. The resistance which has no such component, such as that offered by contracted fibrous tissue.

Frequently the difference between them can only be assessed accurately by repeated movement taken beyond the point at which resistance is first encountered, to feel its characteristics. If pain is severe or if irritability is high it may be impossible to carry out this method of assessment, and full examination of physical resistance is then, quite correctly, not completed. In such a case, as always, a balance must be sought between gaining sufficient information to guide treatment, and avoiding exacerbation of the symptoms by over-examination.

Provided the quality of pain allows (i.e. severity and irritability), repeated movement can be carried beyond the point at which resistance is first encountered. Movement should be of small amplitude at first, increasing from very slow to quick. If this does not give sufficient information, and the state of the joint permits it, the amplitude of the movement can be increased, again beginning slowly and increasing speed with care.

Resistance that is free of muscle activity has the quality of being constant in strength on repeated movement at any given point in the range. In addition, the increase in the strength of the resistance will be in direct proportion to the depth in range, regardless of the speed with which movement is carried out; that is, the resistance felt at one point in movement will always be less than that felt at a point deeper in the range.

It is characteristic of the resistance offered by muscle spasm that it does not show such consistency. Variations in the method of examination produce variations in the quality of the spasm provoked. In particular, the speed of the examining movement is important. The intensity of spasm at any one position will vary according to whether that position is approached quickly or slowly. In addition, the resistance of spasm has a marked quality of recoil, which is less noticeable with spasm-free resistance.

The muscle spasm discussed is the spasm protecting a painful joint but reference must be made briefly to the active muscle contraction affected voluntarily by some patients. This voluntary contraction is frequently out of all proportion to the pain being experienced but may be in direct proportion to an apprehension provoked in the patient if the examiner's technique is poor. Careless or traumatic handling will provoke such a reaction and this will obscure the real clinical findings.

Once the type of resistance has been determined, a range/intensity graph can be plotted for the spasm in the same way as for pain. The method of doing this is now discussed, taking the main types of resistance in turn.

MUSCLE SPASM

As in the case of pain, the intensity and behaviour of muscle spasm is a subjective evaluation. Maximum intensity indicates spasm of a kind which makes the examiner decide to arrest movement, but this is not necessarily of a kind which cannot be overcome. The two may sometimes coincide, but increasing skill and experience will result more and more frequently in maximum spasm being judged to lie well short of intractable resistance. Once again, the student will gain judgment by constantly checking her assessment against that of the experienced physiotherapist.

The joint is moved slowly to the point at which spasm is first elicited, and this point is noted on the base line as S_1. Further movement is then attempted. If maximum intensity is reached before the end of range, spasm thus becomes a limiting factor. This point in the range is noted on the base line by L and S_2 is marked on the upper horizontal (CD) vertically above L.

The graph for the behaviour of spasm is plotted between S_1 and S_2. It will be found that muscle spasm which limits range always reaches its maximum quickly, and thus occupies only a small part of the range measured along AB. Therefore, it will always be depicted as a near-vertical line. *Figure A1.8a* shows spasm which has a little 'give' before maximum is reached. *Figure A1.8b* shows spasm which, when immediately felt, is judged to be of a kind to prohibit all further movement. In some instances when the joint condition is less severe, a little spasm which increases slightly but never prohibits full movement may be felt just before the end of range. In such case there is no point L, and S_2 lies on the vertical line BD (*Figure A1.8c*).

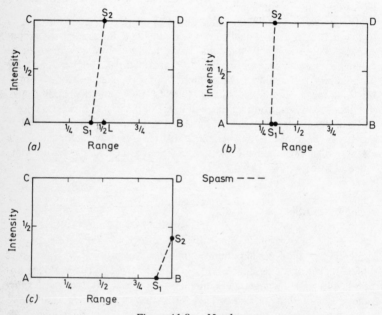

Figure A1.8. – Muscle spasm

SPASM-FREE RESISTANCE

Resistances free of spasm are plotted between points called R_1 and R_2 in a way similarly described for spasm and pain. There are some kinds of spasm-free resistance which cannot be overcome without the use of force, and maximum intensity will here be an objective limitation of movement. In other examples the resistance is of a quality which could be overcome if the movement were taken further and here, maximum intensity indicates a subjective limit imposed by the examiner.

The graphs for spasm-free resistance offer more variation than those for spasm, though not as much as those for pain. There is a hard bone-to-bone feel in which resistance suddenly limits all movement beyond the point at which it is encountered and thus appears as a near-vertical line (*Figure A1.9a*). The resistance may have a softer feel, thus occupying a greater span in the range. In this case it may increase slowly at first and then more quickly as a curved line (*Figure A1.9b*), or it may increase evenly throughout, being depicted as a sloping line (*Figure A1.9c*). If the resistance is never of such an intensity as to prevent full range, there will be no point L and its graph will intersect the vertical BD at R_2 (*Figure A1.9d*).

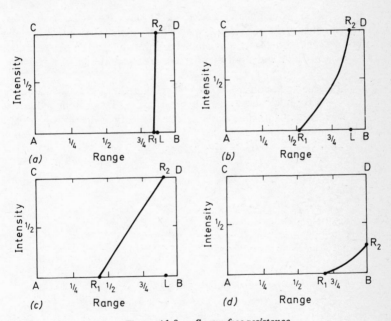

Figure A1.9. – Spasm-free resistance

Appendix 2

The routine by which pain, resistance and muscle spasm are determined and combined in a movement diagram is now described. It will be supposed that elbow extension which is painless at rest is being examined, and that both pain and physical resistance are encountered on movement.

1. The first practical step is to examine the movement carefully and to judge at which point pain begins. This is done by slowly extending the elbow and asking the patient to say when pain

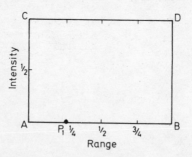

Figure A2.1. – Compiling a movement diagram

starts, and then using oscillatory movements to determine P_1. The information is recorded on the base of the diagram as described in Appendix 1. In this example, pain is first felt at about quarter range (P_1, *Figure A.2.1*).

2. Provided pain is not too severe nor the joint disorder too
    irritable, a slow movement of elbow extension beyond P_1 is
    carried out with the intention of being able to reach the limit
    of the range of extension, i.e. the point B. In our example
    the physiotherapist decides to stop movement at three-quarter
    range and the point L is marked approximately on the base
    line AB (*Figure A2.2*).

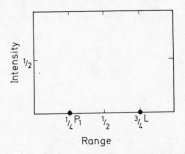

*Figure A2.2. – Compiling a movement
diagram*

3. The next step is to decide exactly why movement was arrested
    at L; that is, which factor or factors were judged to be of
    sufficient intensity at this point in the range for the examiner
    to limit further movement. The diagram is marked accordingly
    on the upper horizontal (vertically above L) by P_2, R_2 or S_2
    to indicate that it was pain, spasm-free resistance, or muscle
    spasm which limited the movement. In the example, R_2 appears
    vertically above L (*Figure A2.3*).

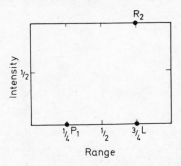

*Figure A2.3. – Compiling a movement
diagram*

4. The most important factor to be kept in mind throughout the examination, assessment and treatment is the behaviour of the patient's pain. Therefore the fourth step is to mark on the vertical line between L and R_2, the intensity of the pain. This assessment of P_2 is made purely subjectively by the physiotherapist. She relates her assessment of the patient's pain to what she considers to be the maximum pain. Then, relating her assessment to 50 per cent of that maximum, she marks P_2 on the vertical line LR_2 either above or below the 50 per cent mark (*Figure A2.4*).

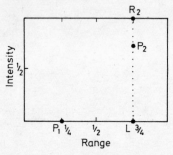

Figure A2.4. – Compiling a movement diagram

5. As pain is such an important factor the next step is for the physiotherapist to move the joint through the range from P_1 to L (with the minimum number of movements) both to assess the behaviour of the pain between P_1 and P_2 and to record the findings on the movement diagram (*Figure A2.5*).

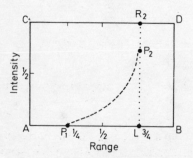

Figure A2.5. – Compiling a movement diagram

6. The point in the range where the limiting factor (resistance) is first encountered is assessed next. Then its behaviour throughout the movement from R_1 to R_2 is assessed and the graph completed. In the example, resistance is first felt at half range, R_1, and rises steeply to maximum intensity at point L (*Figure A2.6*).

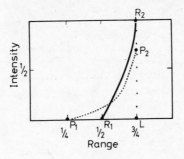

Figure A2.6. – Compiling a movement diagram

7. The last factor to be recorded in the example is a small degree of protective muscle spasm which is felt in the last few degrees of movement. This is recorded between S_1 and S_2, indicating its behaviour between these points (*Figure A2.7*). The movement diagram is now complete.

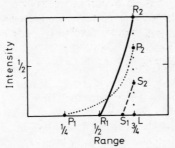

Figure A2.7. – Compiling a movement diagram

A movement diagram may not initially show all the factors which may be present in a particular condition. For example, if the condition is such that the joint is painful even at rest, the examiner might deliberately curb examination. The movement diagram for such a situation might be similar to that shown in *Figure A1.7* (page 343) in which pain alone is plotted. The presence of other factors then remains conjectural (though they may be accurately guessed) since movement is not taken far enough to elicit them.

A more common situation in which all factors may not be shown initially on a movement diagram is when pain and spasm alone appear. For example, in *Figure A2.8*, pain is first provoked at quarter range and rises sharply to a limiting intensity at half range. Intense limiting spasm is also provoked at half range, and thus two factors (P_2 and S_2) appear together on the upper horizontal directly above L. Spasm-free resistance might lie further into the range, but no attempt is made to establish whether or not this is so because of the position and quality of the pain and spasm already provoked. Thus two factors only appear on the diagram.

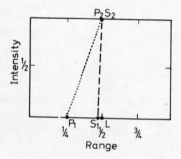

Figure A2.8. – Compiling a movement diagram

The diagram reflects the response of the joint to movement. Because the diagrams show the intensity of factors plotted against their position in range, the response of the joint to different depths of movement can be clearly shown. The speed of movement, on the other hand, is not depicted and something further should be said on this subject.

Increased speed of movement may have the effect of provoking pain and spasm earlier in the range and may also increase their intensity. In addition, speed may affect the extent of the spasm. For example, spasm may be provoked in the deep muscles around a joint at a certain position in range which has a consistent minimum response, in that it cannot be lessened, no matter how this examining movement is modified. It may, however, be very easy to increase this spasm if movement is jerky and awkward. This increase may be shown not only by the spasm being provoked earlier in the range but also by extension of the spasm to other more superficial muscles. As the condition improves, the liability of spasm to increase with quick movements will diminish, and this itself is a measure of progress. Therefore, in the early stages of treatment it would be important to minimize spasm whereas it may be useful later to provoke it by carefully controlled movements, in order to assess its response.

In this regard a slow movement of small amplitude, which is correct examination for one joint, may amount to under-examination of a second; conversely, quicker examining movements which are perfectly judged for the second joint may amount to gross over-examination of the first. What is needed is to match the type of movement used in examination to the condition of the joint. A similar matching of movement to joint condition is required in treatment.

The complexity and subjectivity of the aspects of examination discussed here make them extremely difficult to learn, but unless they are learned the handling of joints does not reach a high standard. Movement diagrams provide a method of gaining insight into the way these factors control, and are controlled by, the skilled use of movement both in examination and treatment. Diagrams are to joint movement what maps are to surface contours.

Index

Accessory movements in examination, 20
Acetabulum, 203
Acromioclavicular joint, 104–107
  anteroposterior movement, 105
  examination, 104
  longitudinal movement, 107
  pain in, 120
  postero-anterior movement, 106
Active movements in examination, 16
Ankle joint, 272–286
  examination, 273, 274, 310
  quick tests, 273
  special tests, 274
  techniques,
    anteroposterior movement, 281
     variations, 282
    dorsiflexion, 277
    eversion, 279
    inversion, 278
    lateral rotation, 284
    longitudinal movement caudad, 285
    longitudinal movement cephalad, 285
    medial rotation, 283
    plantar flexion, 275
    postero-anterior movement, 279
     variations, 281
Arm, flexion of, 21
Arthritis, traumatic, treatment of, 55
Assessment,
  assisting in differential diagnosis, 43

Assessment, (cont.)
  behaviour of pain and, 33, 35
  definitions of, 33
  end of treatment, at, 41
  initial examination, at, 34
  joint stiffness and, 35
  'normality', 43
  objective, 38
  related to pathology, 42
  retrospective, 40
  subjective, 38
  treatment, during, 36
    beginning of each session, at, 37
    between techniques, 39
    during performance, 38
  treatment, for, 32, 334

Calcaneocuboid joint, 297
Capitate, pain in, 22
Carpal bones, 169, 170, 174
Carpal tunnel syndrome, 177
Carpometacarpal joints, 178–181
  accessory movements, 180
  distraction and compression, 181
  examination, 178
  extension, 179
  flexion, 180
  rotation of, 181
  thumb, of, 198, 199, 201
  treatment, 181

Carpus, movement on radius, 165
Chin movement, 324
Compression, effect on weight-bearing
    joints, 17
Costal joints, 315–317
    anteroposterior movement, 316
    examination, 315
Coughing, 317
Cricoid cartilage, 317

Diagnosis,
    assessment related to, 34, 43
    influencing technique, 45

Elbow,
    tennis, 149
    trauma to, 147
Elbow joint, 121–136 (*see also*
        Humero-ulnar joint, Radio-
        humeral joint *and* Superior
        radio-ulnar joint)
    chronic minor pain, 150
    examination of, 121, 122
        general, 151
    pain in, 121
    quick tests, 122
    special tests, 122, 126
    stiffness, 150
    techniques,
        extension, 128
        extension/abduction, 125
        extension/adduction, 122
        flexion, 130
            with accessory movement,
                132
            with longitudinal caudad
                movement, 134
        flexion/abduction and flexion/
                adduction, 126, 132, 133
        longitudinal caudad movement
                (90 degrees flexion), 135
    treatment of, 149
Examination, 7–27, 45, 47, 353
    accessory movements, 20
    assessment of range of movement,
            26
    history taking, 10, 11
    initial,
        assessment at, 34
        diagnosis related to assessment,
            34

Examination, (*cont.*)
    irritability, 9, 14
    joint signs, 15
        compression in, 17
    movement diagram, 26, 338
    objective, 14–18
        general plan of, 25
    other joints, 18
    pain, of, 7, 17
        area of, 7
        behaviour of, 8
        movement aggravating, 9
        nature of, 7
        source of, 13
        variation in, 9
    passive movements, 18
    planning of, 12
    quick tests, 14
    static tests, 18
    subjective, 7–12
        active movements, 16
        initial questions, 8
        summary of, 12
    variation in pressure in, 24

Femur, displacement of head, 216
Fingers, 178 (*see also under specific
        joints*)
Foot (*see also* Ankle joint, Intertarsal
        joint, Tarsometatarsal joint
        and Intermetatarsal joint)
    adduction, 287
    examination of, 310
    interphalangeal joints, 312
    inversion, 286
    medial rotation, 287
    metatarsophalangeal joints, 312
    pain in, 310, 312
    plantar flexion, 287
    stiffness in, 312
    trauma to, 271
Fractures, treatment following, 57
Frozen shoulder, 113
    first stage, 113
    second stage, 114
    third stage, 116

Gait,
    ankle lesions, in, 273
    intertarsal movement and, 288
    knee lesions and, 230

Glenohumeral joint, 62–99, 117
  examination of, 35, 62
    abduction test, 57, 64, 65
    accessory movements, 69
    flexion test, 64, 68
    hand behind back test, 65
    horizontal flexion, 69
    locking position, 66
    objective, 62
    quadrant, 67
    quick tests, 64
    rotator cuff test, 65
    special tests, 65
    subjective, 64
  examination of elbow joint, in,
    123, 124
  fractures of humerus and, 57
  osteoarthritis, 4, 117
  range of movement, 48
  techniques, 69
    abduction, 72
      grade II, 72
      grades III and IV, 74
    anteroposterior movement,
      arm by side, 96
      in abduction, 97
      in horizontal flexion, 97
    flexion and quadrant, 69
      grade II, 69
      grade III, 71
      grade IV, 72
    hand behind back, 80
    horizontal extension, 84
    horizontal flexion, 81
      grades II and III, 82
      grade IV, 83
    lateral movement,
      arm by side, 98
      in flexion, 99
    lateral rotation, 76
    locking position, 75
    longitudinal movement caudad,
      85
      arm by side, 85
      in abduction, 87
      in abduction prone, 88
      in full flexion, 90
      in 90 degrees flexion, 89
    medial rotation, 78
      grade II, 78
      grade IV, 79

Glenohumeral joint (cont.)
  techniques (cont.)
    postero-anterior movement, 91
      in abduction, 94
      in abduction prone, 94
      in flexion, 95
  treatment, 69
    assessment during, 60

Hallux valgus, 313
Hamate, pain in, 22
Hand, bones of, 169
  strains and sprains, 177
Heel, inversion, 286
Heel tap, 271
Hip joint, 203–230
  examination, 203
  pain in, treatment, 229
  quick tests, 204
  special tests, 204
    flexion/adduction, 205
  stiffness of, treatment, 229
  techniques,
    abduction, 225
      in extension, 227
      in flexion, 226
    anteroposterior movement, 225
    extension, 228
    extension/abduction, 227
    flexion/adduction, 207, 229
    lateral movement, 215
    lateral rotation, 213
      in extension prone, 215
      in flexion supine, 214
    longitudinal movement caudad,
      218
      alternative method, 219, 220
      in flexion, 220
    longitudinal movement cephalad,
      222
    medial rotation, 208, 229
      grades I and II, 209
      in extension prone, 212
      in extension supine, 211
      in flexion, 213
    postero-anterior movement, 223
  treatment, 229
Hopping,
  ankle joint lesions, in, 273
  intertarsal movement and, 288

358   INDEX

Humero-ulnar joint,
   examination, 127
   techniques,
      extension, 128
         grade II, 128
         grade III, 129
         grade IV, 130
      flexion, 130
         with accessory movement,
           132
         with longitudinal caudad
           movement, 134
      flexion/abduction, 133
      flexion/adduction, 132
      longitudinal caudad movement
         (90 degrees flexion), 135
Humerus, fractures of, 57, 119
Hyoid bone, movement of, 318
Hyoid joints, 317–318
Hypermobility, treatment of, 56

Inferior radio-ulnar joint, 152–156,
   158, 184
   examination, 152, 153
   quick tests, 153
   special tests, 153
   techniques,
      compression, 155
      longitudinal movement caudad,
         156
      longitudinal movement cephalad,
         156
      postero-anterior and antero-
         posterior movements, 154
Inferior tibiofibular joint, 261–271
   examination, 263, 264
   quick tests, 264
   special tests, 264
   techniques,
      anteroposterior movement, 266
         variation in, 267
         with compression, 267
      compression, 269
      heel tap, 271
      postero-anterior movement,
         264
         variations in, 267
         with compression, 265
      rotation, 270
      treatment, 271
Inflammation, 5

Intercarpal movement, 169–177
   examination, 157, 169, 171
   quick tests, 170
   special tests, 170
   techniques, 170
      anteroposterior movement, 174
      horizontal extension, 170
      horizontal flexion, 172
      longitudinal movement caudad,
         174
      longitudinal movement cephalad,
         175
      pisiform movement, 175
      postero-anterior movement, 173
   treatment, 177
Intercostal movement, 315–317
Intermetacarpal movement, 181–187
   examination, 182
   techniques,
      compression, 186
      general horizontal extension, 185
      general horizontal flexion, 184
      localized horizontal extension,
         186
      localized horizontal flexion, 184
      postero-anterior and antero-
         posterior movement, 186
   treatment, 187
Intermetatarsal movement, 307–310
   examination, 307
   techniques,
      horizontal extension, 309
      horizontal flexion, 308
   treatment, 310
Interphalangeal joints, 187–197
   examination, 187, 188
   of foot,
      examination, 312, 313
      techniques, 313
   quick tests, 187
   techniques,
      abduction, 190
      adduction, 190
      anteroposterior movement, 195
      compression, 194
      distraction, 193
      extension, 189
      flexion, 189
      lateral rotation, 192
      medial rotation, 191
      postero-anterior movement, 194
   treatment, 197

Intertarsal movement, 286–302
  examination, 287, 288, 289
  quick tests, 288
  special tests, 288
  techniques,
    abduction, 297
    adduction, 298
    dorsiflexion, 290, 300
    eversion, 294
      grade III+, 295
      grade IV+, 296
    gliding movements, 302
    inversion, 290
      grade III+, 291
      grade IV+, 292
    plantar flexion, 299
    postero-anterior and antero-
      posterior movements, 301
Irritability, 9, 14
  progress assessment and, 10

Jaw, movements of, 318 (*see also*
  Temporomandibular joint)
Joint pain, treatment of, 47
Joint signs, 6, 15
  comparable, 15
  compression in eliciting, 17
Joint stiffness,
  assessment of, 46
  behaviour of, assessment and, 35
  combined with pain, treatment of,
    48, 51
  resistance in, 36
  treatment of, 50
  variations in, 36
Joints,
  range and pain, 6
  stiff painless, restoring range of, 5

Knee, 230–257 (*see also* Tibiofemoral
  joint *and* Patellofemoral joint)
  composite joint, 261
  examination, 261, 262
  extension, treatment by, 248
  flexion of, 340
    tests of, 231
    treatment, in, 250
  pain in treatment of, 249

Laryngeal joints, 317–318
Loose bodies in joints, repositioning,
  55

Mandible, movements of, 318 (*see also*
  Temporomandibular joint)
Manipulation,
  definitions of, 3
  procedures, 4
  role of, 4
  under anaesthesia, 4
Menisci, displaced, 247
Metacarpal bones, 169
Metacarpophalangeal joints, 187–197
  examination, 187, 188
  quick tests, 187
  techniques,
    abduction, 190
    adduction, 190
    anteroposterior movement, 195
    compression, 194
    distraction, 193
    extension, 189
    flexion, 189
    lateral rotation, 192
    medial rotation, 191
    postero-anterior movement, 194
  treatment, 197
Metatarsalgia, 314
Metatarsophalangeal joints, 312
  examination, 313
  techniques of, 313
  treatment, 314
Mill's manipulation, 149
Mobilization,
  definition, 3
  role of, 4
  symbols of, 336
Movement diagram, 26, 338
  compilation, 339, 348
  muscle spasm in, 345, 348
  pain in, 340, 348
  pain resistance and muscle spasm
    in, 348
  physical resistance in, 344
  resistance in, 348
  spasm-free resistance in, 346
Movements,
  active, 16
  grades of, 29, 336
  increased speed of, 352

Movements, (cont.)
    limitation of due to pain, 46
    normality in, 43
    passive, 18, 20
    range of, assessment of, 26
    regularity in, 30
    resistance to, 344
    types of, 3
Muscle spasm, 47, 338, 345
    behaviour of, 346
    movement diagram, in, 348
    recording, 351
    resistance and, 345
    treatment of, 53
Muscle spasm-free resistance, 346

Navicular-medial cuneiform joint, 298
Normality, 43

Osteoarthritis, 117
    assessment in, 42
    pain in, 6
    treatment of, 55
Osteoarthrosis,
    pain in, 56
    treatment of, 55

Pain,
    accompanied by stiffness, treatment of, 51
    aggravated by movement, 9
    areas of, search for, 7, 8
    assessment of, 334
    behaviour of, 8, 33, 35, 45, 341
        assessment and, 33, 35
        effect on treatment, 33
        recording, 350
    discussion of, 338
    examination of, 7, 17, 24, 340
    frozen shoulder, in, 115
    irregular increase of, 342
    kinds of, 35
    limiting movement, 46
    non-limiting, 343
    normality in, 43
    osteoarthrosis, in, 56
    relief of, 5
    resistance and, 344
    rest, at, 343, 344
    source of, 13

Pain, (cont.)
    treatment of, 47
        combined with stiffness, 48
        with muscle spasm, 53
    variation in, 9, 334
Painful joints, testing for, 6
Painless joints, restoring range of, 5
Passive movements,
    examination, in, 18
    need for relaxation in testing, 20
Patellofemoral joint, 250–257
    examination, 251
    quick tests, 252
    special tests, 252
    techniques,
        compression, 252
        distraction, 256
        longitudinal movement caudad, 254
        transverse movements laterally, 254
        transverse movements medially, 253
    treatment of, 257
Pathology,
    assessment related to, 42
    treatment related to, 55
Physical resistance, 344
Pisiform movement, 175
Pressure, variations in during examination, 24

Quick tests, 14

Radial deviation, 163
Radiocarpal joint, 156
    examination, 159
    quick tests, 157
    special tests, 157
    techniques,
        extension, 162
        flexion, 161
        pronation, 164
        supination, 163
Radiohumeral joint, 147–150
    chronic minor pain of, 150
    examination, 147, 148
    stiffness, 150
    treatment of, 149
Radio-ulnar joint, inferior (see Inferior radio-ulnar joint)

Radio-ulnar joint, superior (*see*
        Superior radio-ulnar joint)
Radius,
    fractures of, 177
    movement on carpus, 165
Recording, 333–337
Recurrences, 42
Relaxation, need for, 20, 28, 29, 30,
        149
Resistance, 344
    movement diagram, in, 348
    muscle spasm and, 345
    recording, 351
    spasm-free, 346
    stiff joints, in, 36
Rheumatoid arthritis, 45
    inflammation in, 5
    treatment of, 55
Rotator cuff test, 65

Scapulothoracic movement,
    elevation and depression, 102
    examination, 100
    protraction, 101
    retraction, 102
    rotation, 103
Shoulder,
    flexion, examination of, 19
    frozen (*see* Frozen shoulder)
    minimal intermittent minor pain,
        118
    painfully stiff, 116
Shoulder girdle, 61–120 (*see also under
        specific joints*)
    quick tests, 61
    special tests, 62
    treatment of, 112
Spasm-free resistance, 346
Squatting,
    ankle joint lesions, in, 273
    knee injury, in, 252
    knee lesions, in, 230
Static tests, 18
Sternoclavicular joint, 108–110
    anteroposterior movement, 109
    compression and distraction, 111
    examination, 108
    pain in, 120
    postero-anterior movement, 110
Stiffness of joints (*see* Joint stiffness)

Superior radio-ulnar joint,
    examination, 137
    techniques,
        anteroposterior movement, 142
            in pronation, 143
            in supination, 142
        longitudinal movement caudad,
            145
        longitudinal movement cephalad,
            146
        postero-anterior movement, 144
            in pronation, 145
            in supination, 144
        pronation, 140
        supination, 138
Superior tibiofibular joint, 257–261
    examination, 258
    techniques,
        anteroposterior movement, 259,
            261
        longitudinal movement cephalad
            and caudad, 260
        postero-anterior movement, 259,
            261
    treatment of, 261
Supraspinatus tendonitis, 112
Swallowing, 317

Tarsometatarsal joints, 289, 298,
        303–306
    examination, 303
    techniques,
        accessory movements, 306
        extension, 304
            alternative method, 305
        flexion, 304
        gliding, 306
        postero-anterior and antero-
                posterior movements, 306
        rotation, 306
        transverse movements, 306
Techniques,
    application of, 45–57
    diagnosis influencing, 45
    positions adopted, 28
    principles of, 28–32
        grades of movement, 29
        intentions, 32
        starting positions, 28, 31
        time factors, 32

Temporomandibular joint, 21, 318–329
examination, 319
locked, 327
pain in, 328
techniques,
depression, 325, 329
lateral chin movement, 324
longitudinal movement caudad,
326
longitudinal movement cephalad,
327
postero-anterior movement, 322
protraction, 322
retraction, 323
transverse movement laterally,
321
transverse movement medially,
320
treatment, 327
Tennis elbow, 149
Thumb, 197–202
carpometacarpal joints, 198, 199,
201
examination of, 198
quick tests, 197
techniques,
adduction, abduction and
opposition, 200
compression, 200
extension, 199
flexion, 199
postero-anterior movement, 201
treatment, 201
Thyroid cartilage, 318
Tibia, rotation of, 243
Tibiofemoral joint, 230–250
examination, 230, 232
quick tests, 230
special tests, 231
techniques,
abduction and adduction, 237
anteroposterior movement, 238,
249
in flexion, 239
extension, 235
extension/abduction, 233
extension/adduction, 235
flexion/abduction, 236
flexion/adduction, 237
lateral movement, 242, 249
lateral rotation, 246
longitudinal movement caudad,
246

Tibiofemoral joint, (cont.)
techniques, (cont.)
longitudinal movement cephalad,
247, 249
medial movement, 243, 249
medial rotation, 243
in flexion prone, 245
in flexion supine, 244
postero-anterior movement, 239,
249
treatment, 247
Tibiofibular joints (see Inferior and
Superior tibiofibular joints)
Toe, big, metatarsophalangeal joint of,
313
Toes, 303
metatarsophalangeal joints, treatment, 314
Torn structures, replacement of, 55
Tarumatic arthritis, treatment of, 55
Treatment (see also under limbs etc.
involved)
application of techniques, 45–57
assessment, 33, 334
definitions of, 33
assessment at end of, 41
assessment during, 36
beginning of each session, at, 37
between techniques, 39
during performance, 38
behaviour of pain affecting, 33
goals of, 41, 47
hypermobility, of, 56
intention of technique, 32
joint pain, of, 47
joint stiffness, of, 50
loose bodies in joints, of, 55
method and assessment, 32–44
pain and muscle spasm, of, 53
plan of, 333
progressing, assessment of, 10
recent fractures, of, 57
recording, 333
regularity in movement, 30
related to pathology, 55
routines, 48, 50, 52, 53
time factors, 32
torn structures, of, 55

Ulna,
deviation, 162
fractures of, 177

Walking,
   ankle lesions, in, 273
   intertarsal movement and, 288
   knee lesions and, 230
Wrist/hand examination, 183
Wrist joint, 156–169
   examination, 159
   quick tests, 157
   special tests, 157
   techniques,
      anteroposterior movement, 166
      extension (general), 160

Walking, (*cont.*)
   techniques, (*cont.*)
      flexion (general), 160
      lateral transverse movement, 167
      medial transverse movement, 168
      postero-anterior movement, 165
      radial deviation, 163
      radiocarpal extension, 162
      radiocarpal flexion, 161
      radiocarpal pronation, 164
      supination, 163
      ulnar deviation, 162